# Cognitive Behavioral Therapy - Basic Principles and Application Areas

*Edited by Cicek Hocaoglu, Celestino Rodríguez, Débora Areces and Vladimir V. Kalinin*

Published in London, United Kingdom

Cognitive Behavioral Therapy - Basic Principles and Application Areas
http://dx.doi.org/10.5772/intechopen.102251
Edited by Cicek Hocaoglu, Celestino Rodríguez, Débora Areces and Vladimir V. Kalinin

Contributors
Sakiko Ogoshi, Yasuhiro Ogoshi, Tohru Saitoh, Akio Nakai, Yoichi Itoh, Masahiro Wakamatu, Tomoyuki Kanno, Kotoko Tanaka, Himanshu Deepak Mansharamani, Bhavika Mansharamani, Prakash Behere, Amit Nagdive, Deepak Mansharamani, Xiaohong Huang, Xiaohua Li, Heng-Wei Cheng, Cicek Hocaoglu, Yavuz Yilmaz, Vladimir V. Kalinin, Anna A. Zemlyanaya, Igor V. Damulin, Ekaterina A. Fedorenko, Maxim A. Syrtsev



First published in London, United Kingdom, 2023 by IntechOpen
IntechOpen is the global imprint of INTECHOPEN LIMITED, registered in England and Wales, registration number: 11086078, 5 Princes Gate Court, London, SW7 2QJ, United Kingdom

British Library Cataloguing-in-Publication Data
A catalogue record for this book is available from the British Library

Additional hard and PDF copies can be obtained from orders@intechopen.com

Cognitive Behavioral Therapy - Basic Principles and Application Areas
Edited by Cicek Hocaoglu, Celestino Rodríguez, Débora Areces and Vladimir V. Kalinin
p. cm.
Print ISBN 978-1-83969-896-5
Online ISBN 978-1-83969-897-2
eBook (PDF) ISBN 978-1-83969-898-9

For EU product safety concerns:
IN TECH d.o.o., Prolaz Marije Krucifikse Kozulić 3, 51000 Rijeka, Croatia,
info@intechopen.com or visit our website at intechopen.com.

# Meet the editors

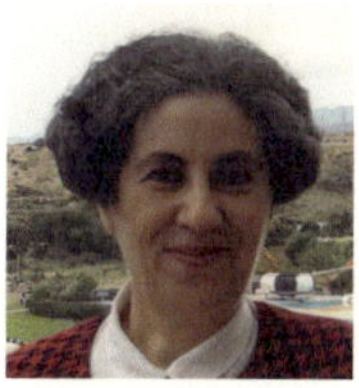

Cicek Hocaoglu obtained her MD from the Faculty of Medicine, Uludag University, Bursa, Turkey. She received postgraduate training in psychiatry at the Faculty of Medicine, Karadeniz Technical University, Trabzon, Turkey. She is currently a Professor and Head of the Department of Psychiatry at the Recep Tayyip Erdogan University Medical School, Rize, Turkey. She has many published national/international scientific articles, book chapters, and congress papers to her credit. Her interests include consultation-liaison psychiatry, suicide, schizophrenia, anxiety disorders, bipolar disorder, and psychopharmacology.

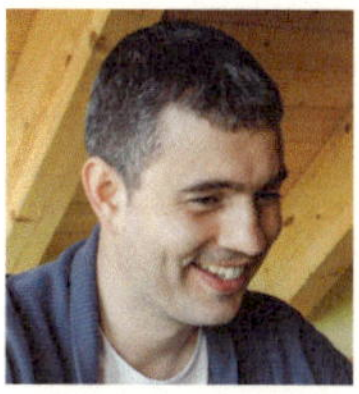

Celestino Rodríguez is a Full Professor in the Department of Psychology and Dean at the Faculty of Teaching Training and Education (University of Oviedo) Spain. His main research areas include learning disabilities, ADHD, and SRL (Self-regulated learning. He is an author of more than 130 papers in peer-reviewed international journals, around 50 chapters, and collaboration in Education, Psychology, and Higher Education books and handbooks. Celestino Rodríguez has made several contributions to national and international conferences (USA, Switzerland, Holland, Italy, Portugal, etc.). He has collaborated with researchers from different countries through different projects and research stays. He is also an Editor of different Journals and a member of the International Association of Research in Learning Disabilities (IARLD).

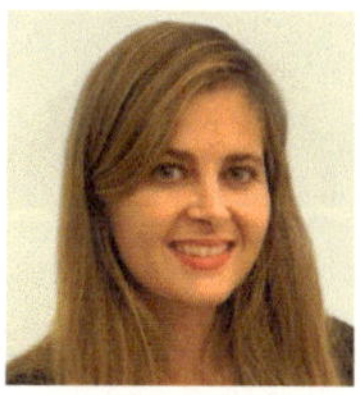

Débora Areces is an Associated Professor in the Department of Psychology of the University of Oviedo, in the area of Education and Developmental Psychology. Her main research areas include Virtual Reality and Neurodevelopmental Disorders. More specifically, her research mainly focuses on the early assessment and intervention of ADHD and learning disabilities from an innovative perspective. She is the author of many articles and parts of books published in both Spanish and English and she has made several contributions to national and international conferences, having taken part in the organizing committee in several of them. Moreover, she has participated in national and European projects related to Learning Disabilities, ADHD and Self-Regulated Learning.

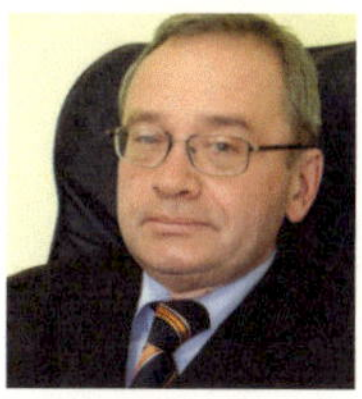

Vladimir V. Kalinin was born in 1952 in a family of physicians in Orenburg (Russian Federation). He graduated from Moscow State Medical Stomatological University (M.D.) in 1976. In 1976-1977 he finished an internship in psychiatry. In 1978 he became a scientific researcher at the Moscow Research Institute of Psychiatry of the Ministry of Health and Social Development where he is still working as Head of the Department. The scope of his scientific interests concerns a broad range of psychiatric problems. The topic of his Doctoral Thesis (1996) concerned anxiety disorders psychopathology and therapy with emphasis on panic disorder. Prof. Kalinin has authored 230 publications, including research articles in professional journals (in Russian and English), three monographs in Russian, and four monographs in English. His biography is included in Marquis's "Who is Who in Medicine and Healthcare" (2006-2007); Who is Who in Science and Engineering 2008-2009"; "Who is Who in the World" (2010, 2011) and in Cambridge International Biographical Centre.

# Contents

# Preface

Neuropsychiatric disorders are among the most common diseases that cause disability worldwide. The etiology, clinical presentation, and treatment of these diseases have been discussed in many studies. There are many psychological, genetic, and environmental risk factors for neuropsychiatric disorders. However, the etiology of neuropsychiatric disorders has not been fully explained yet. In other words, markers for the diagnosis and treatment of neuropsychiatric diseases are not yet available. Difficulties related to etiology and diagnostic evaluations also affect treatment approaches. Because the etiopathogenesis of the diseases is not known exactly, treatment approaches are planned based on existing hypotheses.

Today, psychopharmacological and psychotherapeutic approaches are at the forefront of treatment for neuropsychiatric diseases. Cognitive behavioral therapy (CBT) is the best-known and most-used psychotherapy.

This book includes studies on the psychopathology of neuropsychiatric disorders and CBT. The first section includes two studies examining the role of personality traits in psychopathology. Chapter 1 examines personality traits in children of alcoholic parents. Chapter 2 investigates personality traits investigated as risk factors for the development of cognitive impairment and affective symptomatology in patients with COVID-19.

The second section includes two chapters presenting studies that examine the psychopathology of neuropsychiatric disorders. Chapter 3 examines the use of information and communications technology (ICT) for the individual education support system in neurodevelopmental disorders. Chapter 4 investigates the effects of pregnancy tryptophan fluctuation underlying the ontogenetic origin of neuropsychiatric disorders.

The third section includes one chapter that discusses CBT. Chapter 5 focuses on CBT approaches in the treatment of patients with panic disorder. There are many studies in the literature showing that CBT is 75%–90% effective in the treatment of panic disorder. In the evaluation interviews conducted one year after undergoing CBT, the majority of panic disorder patients maintained their well-being. This chapter explains the cognitive behavioral models and treatment process of panic disorder.

We would like to thank all the authors and publishers who contributed to the preparation of this study for their careful work and hope it will be a valuable resource for our colleagues working in the field of mental health and neurology.

**Cicek Hocaoglu**
Faculty of Medicine,
Department of Psychiatry,
Recep Tayip Erdogan University,
Rize, Turkey

**Celestino Rodríguez**
Full Professor,
Department of Psychology,
University of Oviedo,
Oviedo, Spain

Dean,
Faculty of Teaching Training and Education,
University of Oviedo,
Oviedo, Spain

**Débora Areces**
Associated Professor,
Department of Psychology,
University of Oviedo,
Oviedo, Spain

**Vladimir V. Kalinin**
Department of Organic Brain Disorders and Epilepsy,
Moscow Research Institute of Psychiatry - The Branch
of Serbsky's National Center of Psychiatry and Narcology,
Ministry of Health of Russian Federation,
Moscow, Russian Federation

Section 1

# Personality Traits – The Role in Psychopathology

Chapter 1

# Personality Traits in Children of Alcoholic Parents

*Himanshu Mansharamani, Bhavika Mansharamani, Prakash Behere, Amit Nagdive and Deepak Mansharamani*

## Abstract

Children of alcoholics (COAs) are children who have grown up in families in which either one or both parents are alcoholic. The interplay of several factors such as environmental, cognitive, and genetic vulnerability has been linked to the psychopathology among COAs. The age of elementary school years, i.e., from 6 or 7–15 years of age, is known as the latency developmental period of children, but this phase of development does not apply to COAs, as they are constantly under stress which hinders their self-development. COAs suffer from direct physical, verbal, emotional, and sexual abuse from their alcoholic parent. There is a high need to address the stress to children of persons with substance abuse. Early detection of psychiatric morbidities in such children and appropriate intervention can produce beneficial changes in such children.

**Keywords:** alcohol dependence, children, mental disorders, personality traits, children of alcoholics

## 1. Introduction

Alcohol is a toxic and psychoactive substance with propensity for producing psychological and physical dependence. People since the earliest of times have consumed alcohol for euphoric purposes, to celebrate festivities, to solemnize religious rituals, to grace social functions and to obtain ease from immediate or continuing emotional stress. In today's society, use of alcohol is considered to be a routine part of social environment by many. Although excessive use of alcohol accounts for damage to physical, mental and psychological health, it can be easily overlooked by addicts and their families. Beyond health consequences, excessive alcohol use also causes significant social and economic losses to individuals, their families and society in large.

Among psychoactive substances, most commonly used are caffeine and nicotine, followed by alcohol and cannabis. Excessive alcohol consumption is a major cause of public health concern in most of the countries.

The term alcoholic is associated with 'alcoholism' which is described by the American Medical Association as "A primary, chronic disease with genetic, psychosocial, and environmental factors influencing its development and manifestations. The disease is often progressive and fatal. It is characterized by impaired control over drinking, preoccupation with alcohol, use of alcohol despite adverse consequences, and distortions in thinking, most notably denial. Each of these symptoms may be continuous or periodic" [1].

Alcohol use disorders are among the most prominent psychiatric disorders following a chronic and relapsing course. These are characterized by urge to consume alcohol, loss of control over alcohol intake, compulsive alcohol use, tolerance to quantity of use, withdrawal symptoms and continued alcohol use despite evidence of negative psychological, biological, behavioral, and social consequences [2].

According to the World Health Organization, global attributes of mortality due to alcohol use accounts for about 3 million deaths each year. 5.1% of global burden of disease is attributed to harmful use of alcohol, measured as disability-adjusted life years (DALYs); affecting 7.1% men and 2.2% women. Alcohol is a leading risk factor for disability and premature mortality, accounting for 10% of all deaths among those aged 15–49 years [3]. In 2018, The Global Information System on Alcohol and Health (GISAH) reported that worldwide the total consumption of alcohol amounted to 6.2 liters of ethanol per person aged 15 years and older. Additionally, 26% of the total consumption worldwide is reported as unrecorded consumption. Alcohol consumption also causes harm to the well-being and health of other people around the drinker [4].

Today, alcoholism is clearly seen as a 'Family disease' ravaging not just the individual who drinks excessively but also the entire family. The primary victim is the individual who drinks excessively, but the family members are also affected with just the same intensity, if not more. Excessive drinking by a member in the family affects every member of the family economically, socially and physically and often emotionally and spiritually.

In the United States, the overall lifetime prevalence of alcohol use disorder is around 8% in adolescents and 29% in adults. As reported according to The National Survey of Drug Use and Health in 2019, the prevalence of alcohol use disorder was about 1.7% among adolescents aged 12–17 years, while increasing to 9.3% in those aged 18–25 years [5].

Alcohol use disorders are caused by the interaction of several contributing factors, including, social, cultural, genetic and neurobiological factors. Family and twin studies were the first to show the role of genetics in causation of these disorders. These, followed by adoption studies helped gain clarity over the heritability of these disorders. Studies in the past 35 years report heritability estimates of 40–70% with no sex difference.

Evidence from a recent meta-analysis reported that about 50% of alcohol use disorders are heritable [6].

Although genetic factors play a major role in the etiology of alcohol use disorders, environmental risk factors are also significant. Shared environmental effects are reported to account for ~10% of the variance in alcohol use disorders. A common genetic and environmental risk factor is parental alcohol use disorder. It is estimated that children of alcoholic parents are 3–4 times more likely to develop alcoholism as compared to children of non-alcoholic parents [7]. Gene-environment interactions also contribute to causation and persistence of these disorders. Psychological factors affect genetic vulnerability of developing alcoholism. One of the lesser studied but significant etiological risk factor for alcohol use disorders is temperament or personality traits. Personality characteristics and social environment of an individual interact to contribute in the formation of any kind of problematic behavior [8].

## 2. Temperament and personality

Temperament is defined as an innate biological disposition of how a child reacts behaviourally and emotionally to diverse physiological, psychosocial, and energetic stimuli [9].

Chess and Thomas [10] had introduced the concept of temperament as they described it as the style of behavior (the 'how'). Temperament emerges early in life, and manifests in behaviors during the toddler and preschool period that are viewed as inborn or maturational. Temperamental traits exert an influence on the individuals cognitive and social development. They form the foundation of personality.

Personality on the other hand is described as the content of thought, coping styles, values and beliefs of an individual (the 'what'). Personality emerges later in life and reflects patterns of behavior, emotions, and cognitions that are focused on aspects of self. Personality traits are influences by family, peers and context across development [11].

## 3. Personality traits and alcoholism

Theories of alcoholism propose that the genetic predisposition for alcoholism in children of alcoholic parents is partially mediated by temperament or personality. Temperament and personality traits have consistently been found to be heritable. Several genetic factors have consistently been implicated in contributing to differences in personality traits. A recent meta-analysis states that the average effect of genetic contributions to individual differences in personality is about 40% [12].

Personality traits might represent a common mediating factor for risk of alcoholism in children due to parental history. This may be caused by multiple pathways, two of the important ones being genetics and psychosocial factors. As known, personality is genetically heritable and is also developed by individual experience of psychosocial factors, including development of coping mechanisms and cognitions to deal with stressors. Families of alcoholics vary on a continuum of dysfunction as many other psychological disturbances in parenting, like abuse or neglect can occur with, or as a consequence of parental alcoholism. Contrary to expectation, personality traits in children of alcoholics are highly variable and heterogenous. Thus, familial dysfunction can produce a variety of different consequences on the personality of children of alcoholic parents [13, 14].

Personality disorders (PDs) are defined as "disorders involving pervasive patterns of perceiving, relating to, and thinking about the environment and the self that interfere with long-term functioning of the individual and are not limited to isolated episodes." A personality disorder is persistent and enduring, usually beginning in adolescent or early adulthood, leading to impairment in social and/or occupational functioning [15].

Epidemiological studies have shown an average prevalence of PDs in general population as about 10%, ranging from 4.4% to 21.5% [16].

Personality disorders and substance use disorders are a comorbidity seen more commonly than expected by chance. In individuals with a Personality Disorder, the risk of a comorbid substance use disorder (SUD) is increased by five-to 12-fold, alcohol being a more commonly used substance among others [17].

According to The National Epidemiologic Survey on Alcohol and Related Conditions (NESARC), prevalence of alcohol use disorders (AUD) was found to be 30.3%. The prevalence of PDs in AUDs ranged between 0.5% and 7.9% to [16].

In individuals with AUD, Cluster B personality disorders were more prevalent as compared to Cluster A and C. Identification of distinct personality disorders concluded that borderline personality disorder and antisocial personality disorder are most commonly seen. A positive correlation has also been observed between severity of AUD and co-occurrence of other psychiatric diagnosis along with PDs [18].

## 4. Comorbid personality disorder and substance use disorder

Several hypotheses have been given to explain the common comorbidity of PDs and SUD suggesting that the evidenced corelation between them is not just a coincidental finding.

### 4.1 Primary substance use disorder

This theory postulates that SUDs are the primary disorder contributing to the development of pathological personality traits. Repeated trauma and direct effect of neurobiological changes due to continued substance use may cause personality deviations that appear related to the development of a PD.

### 4.2 Primary personality disorder

Substance abuse can be seen as a secondary effect to the primary diagnosis of a PD. The presence of certain maladaptive personality traits may play a role in the development of substance use disorders, concluding that personality traits are developmental antecedents of alcoholism. The most empirical evidence is present for this model.

Another hypothesis of the cause of secondary substance use in personality disorders is self-medication. Individuals with personality disorders and other comorbid psychiatric disorders are more likely to develop alcoholism as an attempt to escape and self-regulate their unmanageable or unwanted emotions [19, 20].

## 5. Reward pathway

The reward sensitivity or the mesolimbic pathway is a dopaminergic system between ventral tegmental area in the midbrain and the nucleus accumbens in the limbic system. Natural rewards like food, sex and social interaction activates this system thus leading to the feeling of pleasure. This pathway also regards the positively reinforcing properties of substance as a motivating factor.

Neurobiological vulnerability factors such as alteration in this pathway or release of the neurotransmitter dopamine may cause difficulties with impulsivity and impulse control. This may play a crucial role in development and/or maintenance of substance use disorders. Some individuals experience exposure to novelty as rewarding. Other than natural rewards, the reward pathway is activated by novelty as well as by cues predicting their occurrence. This suggests that novelty itself acts as a motivating factor for individuals to explore an environment for potential rewards. Individuals high on traits like reward or novelty seeking are more likely to develop substance use disorders. Longitudinal studies have demonstrated that novelty seeking in childhood and adolescence predicts later substance use problems [21]. Hyperresponsiveness or hypersensitivity to the effects of substances develops more strongly in individuals with a general sensitivity to positive reinforcements [22].

Family studies have shown that even healthy family members of drug-dependent patients are more prone to have impulsive personality traits and shortcomings in executive functioning [23]. A Norwegian twin study suggests that the trait "impulsivity" is a genetic risk factor, and "conduct disorder" resembles a combined genetic and development risk for suffering from AUD. The study also found that "conduct disorder" and "self-harming impulsivity" predicted alcohol use disorder more successfully than diagnoses of PDs [24].

Generally, patients with PDs and comorbid SUDs show certain differences as compared to those without co-occurring SUD. They have a younger age of onset of substance related problems, more frequent use of other illicit substances, more problems with social interactions and poorer psychosocial functioning [25].

## 6. Children of alcoholic parents

Children are vulnerable and easily affected by the environment which is provided to them while growing up. Experiences during the developmental period of life affects the emotional, social and cognitive development and forms the base of behavior and therefore personality in later life. During this period of life, children learn social, adaptive and coping skills to deal with situations. These experiences are generated primarily by parents, other family members, in school and among peers. Successful experiences provide the child with a sense of competence, stable self-identity and coping skills, whereas failure results in a sense of inadequacy, inferiority and poor or maladaptive coping skills.

Not only does alcohol harm the alcoholic, but it also has a negative impact on the family, causing extreme emotional pain and suffering. Out of the many significant costs' alcoholism exacts upon society and the family, one of its most detrimental may be its negative effect upon the children who grow up with alcoholic parents. A child who is forced to stay and grow in a dysfunctional environment is the one who suffers the most. They are directly affected by their parent's drinking problem and indirectly by other factors associated with the familial dysfunction. Several studies have demonstrated an association between problem drinking in parents and negative outcomes in their children.

Vulnerability is defined as "being susceptible to physical harm, damage, emotional injury or attack." It is conceptualized as the experiences that cause stress and anxiety and negatively affect an individual's physiological, psychological, and social functions [26, 27].

Children of alcoholics are affected by a variety of problems throughout their lifespan. They are victims of an alcoholic family environment characterized by disruption, deviant and in-adequate parental roles and parent-child relationship. These variables affect normal child development, emotional regulations and expressions, both acutely and chronically. They tend to experience abuse which can be verbal, physical, emotional and sexual, and neglect in terms of important needs in the areas of child care, safety, health and material wellbeing leading to subsequent mental health and behavioral problems [28–30]. Although a substantial proportion of children also show resilience due to other protective factors [31].

Two broad classes of psychopathological traits and symptoms during childhood have been identified in Children of alcoholics: Internalizing symptoms and Externalizing symptoms. These categories were made to help identify problem behaviors in children and adolescents that underlie the development of psychopathology in adults in later life.

The observation that COAs show increased risk of behavioral disorders, may be due to genetic heritability of pathological traits that are transmitted to them by their alcoholic parents, poor rearing environment provided to them, or a combination of both. Genetic factors by the evidence of adoption and twin studies have more clearly been implicated in the development of alcoholism in children of alcoholic parents, while shared environmental factors have been implicated in the development of psychopathological traits in the absence of alcoholism in these children [32].

The environmental cause for development of these behavioral symptoms is directly due to the effect of parental alcoholism and indirectly due to the disrupted family environment, parental comorbidity and/or genetic predisposition to the development of pathological traits.

Both genetic and environmental risk factors intertwine and interact to increase the risk of psychopathological traits and alcoholism in children of alcoholic parents. Therefore, a stress diathesis model best explains the cause of psychopathology in COAs. A predisposing genetic vulnerability (diathesis) is present in offspring of alcoholic parents, which interacts with the environmental stressors (stress) experienced by them resulting in the development of maladaptive personality traits and even alcoholism in later life.

Internalizing psychopathology includes symptoms of anxiety and depression; while externalizing symptoms encompasses 'acting out' behaviors characterized by inattention, impulsivity, defiance, aggression and violent acts [14]. Studies have also reported that these children are more vulnerable to development of mental disorders, early drug use and dependence, high risk sexual behavior and suicide [33]. They are also at a greater risk to develop guilt, shame, social withdrawal, anxiety and poor academic performance when compared to non-abused children [34].

## 7. Personality characteristics of children of alcoholics

Reports from studies on personality characteristic of COAs are highly variable and heterogenous. This heterogeneity can be explained by the presence of variability within the families of alcoholics and can be understood as a continuum of family dysfunction. Families with alcoholic parents differ in other associated behaviors that contribute to dysfunction, like other psychological disturbances, type of parenting, attachment with non-alcoholic parent, emotional support by other family members, neglect or abuse. These variables influence the consequences on the personality of COAs [14].

Therefore, many studies have described subtypes of personalities instead of specific traits.

Theory and research on classifying subtypes of personalities present in children of alcoholic parents began decades ago.

Four personality styles in COAs were proposed by Wegscheider [35] based on clinical experience:

1. The Enabler (caretaker)—tries to reduce harm to the family through enabling behaviors like taking care or doing things and making excuses for the addict.

2. The Hero—extremely responsible, perfectionist, overachiever, highly stresses, put a lot of pressure on themselves, often workaholics with Type A personalities.

3. The Scapegoat child—acts out, rejected by parents, blamed for all the family problems.

4. The Mascot (Clown)—child uses humor as defense against feeling pain and fear; tries to reduce family stress through humor.

5. The Lost child—quiet, isolated, spends most time in solitary activities, largely neglected by parents, may escape by forming own fantasy world [35].

Four dominant roles that children growing up in an addicted household are likely to acquire, were given by Dr. Claudia Black. These roles are explained to be coping mechanisms developed from underlying fear and insecurities and are typically carried on through adulthood.

1. The Responsible Child—takes responsibility of the family but remains isolated; self-disciplined, organized, perfectionist, inflexible, severe need for control.

2. The Adjuster—flexible, unable to make decisions, unable to initiate.

3. The Placater—takes care of family but unable to care for self, sensitive to others, unable to receive care.

4. The Act-out Child—suffers difficulty expressing needs and relating to others, faces social problems [36].

Although, there is weak empirical evidence for these clinical taxonomies.

In further studies, it was concluded that the presence of these subtypes is not specific to parental alcohol use disorder, rather context variables such as family disruption due to various other factors were a more potent predictor of presence of these subtypes.

Three broad categories of personality traits can be described on the basis of observable behavioral differences in measures of personality.

## 8. Neuroticism/negative emotionality

Children in this category have a tendency to experience negative emotions and affective states, including inability to manage stressful situations, depression, anxiety, propensity to blame oneself, low self-esteem, high levels of guilt feelings and sensitivity to criticism. Children of alcoholics show higher levels of negative emotionality as compared to non-COAs. Neuroticism in COAs is reported to be more common in those with alcoholic parents with comorbid anxiety and depression as compared to those with alcoholic parents without comorbidities.

Additionally, as compared to non-alcoholic COAs, COAs at high risk of alcoholism show higher levels of anxiety [37].

## 9. Impulsivity/disinhibition

This personality dimension is most commonly associated with COAs. Children in this category have a tendency to act before considering future consequences and show traits of sensation and novelty seeking behavior, poor self-control, impulsive behavior and aggressiveness [38]. These traits also predispose them to development of antisocial personality and alcoholism in later life. This suggests that the presence of these characteristics might represent a mediator of genetic heritability of alcoholism in families [39].

On comparison of aggressive behaviors between children of alcoholics and children of non-alcoholics, the later showed lower levels of aggressive behaviors at the age of 18–48 months. Moreover, they showed progressively decreasing levels of aggressive behaviors at the age of 36–48 months [40]. At the age of 2 years children of alcoholics showed more externalizing behaviors and poorer self-regulation as compared to children of non-alcoholics. The ability to self-regulate, that is, inhibitory control is usually developed by the age of 2 years in children. Children of alcoholics show a failure to develop this ability as compared to healthy children. Children in this category also show poor global and adaptive functioning [41].

## 10. Extraversion/sociability

This personality dimension also explained as positive emotionality or affectivity, encompasses traits like sociability, flexibility and gregariousness. This characteristic has not differentiated COAs from non-COAs in research studies. It is understood that sociability may be a positive feature in high functioning and resilient children or it may also be a trait in those with disinhibited behavior [37].

On examining the effect of maternal vs. paternal alcoholism on personality traits of children, it was reported that both maternal and paternal alcoholism is related to temperament and character dimensions in children and adolescents, irrespective of offspring gender. Children of alcoholic fathers are more likely to show novelty seeking as a temperamental trait while those of alcoholic mothers show lower self-directedness as a character dimension [42].

Five distinct personality subtypes were found in adolescent and adult children of alcoholics:

1. Angry/externalizing subtype:

   These adolescents show characteristic features of disturbance of conduct. They are prone to act impulsively, without foresight or regard for consequences. They express intense irritability and anger, out of proportion to the situation. They also show psychopathic features, such as being manipulative and deceitful, lacking empathy for others and taking advantage of them. They experience disruption of childhood attachments, poor functioning in school and poor adaptive functioning. These adolescents show significantly higher rates of substance abuse disorder and antisocial personality disorder. This subtype of adolescents shows features similar to the category of "the scapegoat" described by Wegscheider [35].

2. Awkward/inhibited subtype:

   These adolescents show internalizing problems and deficits in social behavior. These adolescents have a tendency to be passive, avoidant, and depressed. They tend to feel inadequate and inferior. They have difficulty in acknowledging and expressing anger towards other accompanied by fear of rejection or abandonment. They also show the higher rates of avoidant personality disorder and poor functioning in school and social situations. This subtype of adolescents resembles the "Lost Child" as described by Wegscheider [35].

3. Hyper-conscientious/high-functioning subtype:

   These adolescents show a tendency to be conscientious and responsible. They are able to use their abilities to their advantage. They have moral standards and try to live up to them. They tend to be insightful and are able to understand their feeling and empathize with others. This group of adolescents also show higher functioning in school and higher adaptive functioning.

4. Emotionally dysregulated subtype:

   These adolescents show features characterized by intense emotional experiences and unstable relationships. They tend to experience extremes of all emotions, including anxiety, anger and sadness; that tend to change rapidly and unpredictably. They are prone to feeling of emptiness. They have a fear of being rejected or abandoned. They lack a stable sense of self as values, attitudes and feelings about self are derived from external situations. These adolescents show high rates of borderline personality traits.

5. Sexualized/self-defeating:

   These adolescents tend to act impulsively and engage in thrill-seeking and self-mutilating behaviors. They are more prone to abuse alcohol and act promiscuously. They tend to have unstable and abusive relationships.

Adolescents and adults have also reported to be more pessimistic about their future and poor emotional and physical well-being [43].

## 11. Personality characteristics of alcoholic children of alcoholics

Alcoholism in parents is an established risk factor for development of psychopathology and alcoholism in their children. Adoption and twin studies have consistently indicated that genetic factors primarily contribute to development of alcoholism in male offspring of alcoholic parents. While similar studies in women have shown inconsistent findings. This has led to an understanding that genetic risk is a less important etiological factor in the development of alcoholism in female offspring of alcoholic parents [44]. For both men and women, the number of alcoholic parents is directly related to level of psychopathology, with children with both alcoholic parents being at a greater risk. COAs who are more prone to develop alcoholism show higher traits of impulsivity, aggressive behavior, sensation seeking, emotional dysregulation and antisocial behavior since childhood [45].

Few studies have reported that children of alcoholic fathers are more prone to develop alcoholism as compared to children of alcoholic mothers, indicating a stronger influence of paternal alcoholism. Although, a meta-analysis concluded that both groups of children are equally likely to develop alcoholism in later life [32].

Four major personality traits have been reported to strongly predict substance use by children of alcoholics [46].

1. Impulsivity.

2. Sensation seeking.

3. Anxiety sensitivity, and

4. Hopelessness.

Impulsivity and sensation seeking are described above. Anxiety sensitivity can be understood as an unspecific or situation specific fear, and desire to relieve, anxiety symptoms. Hopelessness is considered as a tendency for depression, a general negative perspective of life and low regard of self [47].

Behavioral undercontrol, explained as the traits of impulsivity, nonconformity, rebelliousness and thrill seeking is the most commonly associated personality dimension in alcoholic progeny. Genetic diathesis of alcoholism is said to be partly mediated by the presence of this personality dimension.

Premorbid traits that have been found to be predictive to early onset of alcohol abuse and dependence are those associated with antisocial personality. These include overactivity, poor attention, distractibility, impatience, low empathy and aggressive behavior. Retrospective and longitudinal studies have confirmed that the presence of antisocial or impulsive traits are characteristic of majority of early onset or young alcoholics while only a minority of late onset alcoholics.

It is also suggested that passive-dependent or oral traits including being rigid, tendency to cry easily, being passive and pessimistic are associated with loss of control pattern of drinking and late onset alcoholism.

However, studies have not been able to disentangle the extent to which this personality dimension is related to genetic or environmental risk factors associated with parental alcoholism [48].

## 12. Factors influencing negative impact on children of alcoholics

Various factors contribute to the impact of parental alcoholism in development of negative consequences for their children. Certain factors may minimize or maximize the adverse effects associated with parental alcohol abuse. Several vulnerability and risk factors may increase the negative impact while protective factors may decrease the same by developing resilience. Essentially, these factors play a significant role in moderating the relation between parental problem drinking and negative behavioral and personality outcome in their children.

### 12.1 Age

A survey of college students conducted by Kim and Lee [49] concluded that age was a moderating factor with young children being more negatively affected as compared to adolescents or adults. The survey also reported that as they age, COAs tend to become more insensible to their alcoholic parents [49].

Adult COAs also tend to show decline in the negative outcomes between late 20s and early 30s [50].

### 12.2 Gender

Studies have observed no significant effect of gender in intergenerational transmission of alcoholism by influence of both genetic and environmental factors. Parental alcohol use disorders conferred the same risk for both male and female offspring for development of alcoholism in them [32]. In the context of psycho-pathological traits, females from childhood up till adulthood are more vulnerable to development of internalizing symptoms like depression, anxiety and inability to manage stress. On the other hand, males are more prone to developing externalizing symptoms including aggressive and impulsive behavior [51].

### 12.3 Attachment

Attachment, a concept originated by John Bowlby, is defined as "the emotional tone between children and their caregivers. It is evidenced by an infant's seeking behaviour." A child forms attachment relationship with his or her parents during the first year of life. Attachment is primarily facilitated by the interaction between mother and infant and provides infants with a feeling of security [52]. This serves as a foundation for psychosocial development, personality and formation of future relationships. Secure attachment is developed from a caregiving environment and characterized by parental responsiveness and consistency.

In the context of parental alcoholism, poor mother-child relationship has a deleterious effect on the child's behavior and therefore later personality. On the other hand, secure attachment with mother is considered as a protective factor against the negative impact of father's alcoholism. Studies have indicated that among alcoholic families, infants with secure attachment at the age of 12 months showed fewer externalizing behavior problems at the age of 24-36 months when compared to those with insecure attachment. Toddlers in secure relationships are guided by their supportive caregivers in soothing and managing negative emotions [53]. Children who develop secure attachment are able to understand and self-regulate their emotional responses. Those with insecure attachment either under or over- regulate their emotions leading to development of internalizing or externalizing symptoms. Thus, attachment is a significant moderating factor between paternal alcoholism and child behavior [54].

### 12.4 Cognitive ability

Cognitive ability of children measured by academic performance and school achievement was seen to be lower in children of alcoholics as compared to healthy controls [55]. Poor cognition ability considered as the ability to think, reason and recognize emotions may make the children more vulnerable to be affected by the negative external environment. While, poor academic performance and achievement in school and social setting may also be the result of both poor cognition and negative impact of parental alcoholism.

### 12.5 Temperament

Temperament influences the development of social and cognitive skills in later life. Infants show individualized patterns of reactivity including responsiveness to presence or absence of parents, eating behavior and sleep-wake cycle. On the basis of these, three groups of temperament were formed: easy, difficult and slow to warm up. These individual differences persist into childhood and adolescence and form the basis of personality in later life. Temperamental traits of high activity, poor attention, impulsivity, high emotionality and low self-regulation have been associated with high risk of dysregulated behavior problems in children. The presence of these may also be indicative of maladaptive patterns of behavior and even addiction in later life [56]. Presence of a difficult affective temperament also mediated the relationship between paternal alcoholism and resulting maladjustment in children [57].

Edwards, Eiden, Colder et al. (2006) have also described difficult or negative temperament as a risk factor affecting COAs [55]. While those with flexible or positive temperaments were seen to be more resilient as compared to controls [57].

These temperamental characteristics may be indicative of behavioral dysregulation, and may lay the initial groundwork for later maladaptive developmental patterns and even addiction [56].

### 12.6 Family environment

Family discord, marital conflict and violence in addition to parental alcoholism are important mediating factors in affecting the child's personality and behavior. Unresponsive, inconsistent and violent behavior by drinking parents is associated with poor family functioning thus causing low self-esteem and maladaptive patterns in children [13].

Comorbid psychopathology in drinking parents is another factor influencing problem behaviors in children of alcoholics. Presence of comorbid psychiatric illness with alcoholism in parents puts their children at a greater risk as compared to those whose parents do not have comorbid disorders. Mental health of parents significantly affects the psychology of children regardless of their alcohol use. Studies have reported that the presence of maternal depression in families with alcoholic fathers increased the risk of development of internalizing problems in children.

In a study by Hussong et al. [58] three types of families: antisocial alcoholic families, depressed alcoholic families, and alcoholic only-families, were compared. It was concluded that children from both antisocial-alcoholic families and depressed-alcoholic families showed increased risk above that shown by children in alcoholic-only families [58].

In conclusion, these vulnerability and protective factors can be useful in development of preventive strategies and interventions for children of alcoholic parents. This may help in reducing the impact of negative outcomes and promoting emotional well being in them.

## 13. Summary

Alcoholism is a prominent problem in today's world and alcohol misuse is a common lifestyle-related cause of physical and mental disorders. Problem drinking is a serious problem in itself but it also affects other people as those who engage in drinking are parents and family members to others. Parental alcoholism negatively affects their children not only directly but also indirectly due to the associated behaviors contributing to inconsistent pattern of parenting, neglect, abuse and violence. Children of those with comorbid psychological or psychiatric disorders along with alcoholism are seen to be more at risk. Children are vulnerable to the deleterious effects of such environment, acutely during their growing up years and also chronically until adulthood. Genetic factors are also implicated in contributing to development of risk-personality and future alcoholism. Children of alcoholics are reported to show more internalizing and externalizing symptoms during childhood. As they grow, these symptoms and traits crystalise to form maladaptive patterns of behavior.

Although, a homogenous group of personality traits have not been reported, several traits have been associated with children of alcoholics. Impulsivity, disinhibited behavior and negative emotionality are the most commonly associated subtypes seen in children of alcoholics. Evidence also suggests that common genetic factors may underlie the development of both the personality traits and alcoholism. They have poor self-regulation in childhood and later self-control, inability to deal with negative emotions and higher levels of aggression as compared to children of non-alcoholic parents.

Research focusing on these characteristic personality traits as endophenotypes in alcoholism should provide with better preventive strategies.

## Author details

Himanshu Mansharamani[1*], Bhavika Mansharamani[2], Prakash Behere[3], Amit Nagdive[4] and Deepak Mansharamani[5]

1 LNCT Medical College and JK Hospital, Bhopal, Madhya Pradesh, India

2 LNCT Medical College and Sevakunj Hospital, Indore, Madhya Pradesh, India

3 CAMHS, Raigmore Hospital, Inverness, Scotland

4 CNTW Mental Health Trust, Morpeth, Northumberland, UK

5 Gokuldas Hospital, Indore, Madhya Pradesh, India

*Address all correspondence to: himanshu.mansha@gmail.com

## References


[1] Morse R. The definition of alcoholism. Journal of the American Medical Association. 1992;**268**(8):1012

[2] American Psychiatric Association. Diagnostic and Statistical Manual of Mental Disorders. 5th ed. Arlington, VA: American Psychiatric Association; 2013

[3] World Health Organization. Global Status Report on Alcohol and Health 2018. Geneva: WHO; 2018

[4] Global Information System on Alcohol and Health. Who.int. 2022. Available from: https://www.who.int/data/gho/data/themes/global-information-system-on-alcohol-and-health

[5] Abuse S. Key substance use and mental health indicators in the United States: Results from the 2019 National survey on drug use and health. FIU Digital Commons. 2022. Available from: https://digitalcommons.fiu.edu/srhreports/health/health/32/

[6] Verhulst B, Neale MC, Kendler KS. The heritability of alcohol use disorders: A meta-analysis of twin and adoption studies. Psychological Medicine. 2015;**45**(5):1061-1072

[7] Obot IS, Wagner FA, Anthony JC. Early onset and recent drug use among children of parents with alcohol problems: Data from a national epidemiologic survey. Drug and Alcohol Dependence. 2001;**65**(1, 1):-8

[8] Carvalho AF, Heilig M, Perez A, Probst C, Rehm J. Alcohol use disorders. The Lancet. 2019;**394**(10200):781-792

[9] Kagan J et al. Galen's Prophecy. Boulder: Basic Books; 1998

[10] Chess S, Thomas A. Temperament in Clinical Practice. New York: Guilford; 1986

[11] Rothbart MK. Becoming Who We Are: Temperament and Personality in Development. New York: Guilford Press; 10 Jun 2011

[12] Vukasović T, Bratko D. Heritability of personality: A meta-analysis of behavior genetic studies. Psychological Bulletin. 2015;**141**(4):769-785

[13] Lease SH. A model of depression in adult children of alcoholics and nonalcoholics. Journal of Counseling & Development. 2002;**80**:441-451

[14] Sher KJ. Psychological characteristics of children of alcoholics. Alcohol Health and Research World. 1997;**21**(3):247-254

[15] APA. Diagnostic and Statistical Manual of Mental Disorders. 5th ed. Wahington, DC: American Psychiatric Publishing (DSM-5); 2013

[16] Hasin D, Grant B. The national epidemiologic survey on alcohol and related conditions (NESARC) Waves 1 and 2: Review and summary of findings. Social Psychiatry and Psychiatric Epidemiology. 2015;**50**(11):1609-1640

[17] Trull TJ, Jahng S, Tomko RL, Wood PK, Sher KJ. Revised NESARC personality disorder diagnoses: Gender, prevalence, and comorbidity with substance dependence disorders. Journal of Personality Disorders. 2010;**24**(4):412-426

[18] Barral C, Daigre C, Bachiller D, Calvo N, Ros-Cucurull E, Gancedo B, et al. Severity factors associated with borderline personality disorder among misusers in an outpatient sample in Spain. Journal of Addictive Diseases. 2017;**36**(2):93-96

[19] Khantzian EJ. The self-medication hypothesis of addictive disorders: Focus on heroin and cocaine dependence. The American Journal of Psychiatry. 1985;**142**(11):1259-1264

[20] Khantzian EJ. Understanding addictive vulnerability: An evolving psychodynamic perspective. Neuropsychoanalysis: An Interdisciplinary Journal for Psychoanalysis and the Neurosciences. 2003:5-21

[21] Cloninger CR, Sigvardsson S, Bohman M. Childhood personality predicts alcohol abuse in young adults. Alcoholism, Clinical and Experimental Research. 1988;**12**:494-505

[22] Zuckerman M. Behavioral Expressions and Biosocial Bases of Sensation Seeking. New York: Cambridge University Press; 24 Jun 1994

[23] Ersche KD, Turton AJ, Chamberlain SR, Müller U, Bullmore ET, Robbins TW. Cognitive dysfunction and anxious-impulsive personality traits are endophenotypes for drug dependence. American Journal of Psychiatry. 2012;**169**(9):926-936

[24] Rosenström T, Torvik FA, Ystrom E, Czajkowski NO, Gillespie NA, Aggen SH, et al. Prediction of alcohol use disorder using personality disorder traits: A twin study. Addiction. 2018;**113**(1):15-24

[25] Langås AM, Malt UF, Opjordsmoen S. In-depth study of personality disorders in first-admission patients with substance use disorders. BMC Psychiatry. 2012;**12**(1):1

[26] The American Heritage Dictionary. The American Heritage Dictionary of the English Language. 5th ed. Boston, MA: Houghton Mifflin Company; 2012

[27] De Santis J. Exploring the concepts of vulnerability and resilience in the context of HIV infection. Research and Theory for Nursing Practice. 2008;**22**(4):273-287

[28] Solis MJ, Shadur MJ, Burns RA, Hussong MA. Understanding the diverse needs of children whose parents abuse substances. Current Drug Abuse Reviews. 2012;**5**(2):135-147

[29] Jose J, Cherayi S. Effect of parental alcohol abuse severity and child abuse and neglect on child behavioural disorders in Kerala. Child Abuse and Neglect. 2020;**107**:104608

[30] Jaisoorya TS, Beena KV, Ravi GS, Thennarasu K, Benegal V. Alcohol harm to adolescents from others' drinking: A study from Kerala, India. Indian Journal of Psychiatry. 2018;**60**(1):90

[31] Wlodarczyk O, Schwarze M, Rumpf H, Metzner F, Pawils S. Protective mental health factors in children of parents with alcohol and drug use disorders: A systematic review. PLoS One. 2017;**12**(6):e0179140

[32] Slutske W, D'Onofrio B, Turkheimer E, Emery R, Harden K, Heath A, et al. Searching for an environmental effect of parental alcoholism on offspring alcohol use disorder: A genetically informed study of children of alcoholics. Journal of Abnormal Psychology. 2008;**117**(3):534-551

[33] Norman RE, Byambaa M, De R, Butchart A, Scott J, Vos T. The long-term health consequences of child physical abuse, emotional abuse, and neglect: A systematic review and meta-analysis. PLoS Medicine. 2012;**9**(11):e1001349

[34] Manton E, MacLean S, Laslett AM, Room R. Alcohol's harm to others: Using

qualitative research to complement survey findings. International Journal of Alcohol and Drug Research. 2014;**3**(2):143-148

[35] Wegscheider S. Another Chance: Hope and Health for the Alcoholic Family. Palo Alto, CA: Science and Behavior Books; 1981

[36] Black C. Children of alcoholics, alcohol, health and research. World. 1979;**4**:23-27

[37] Berkowitz A, Perkins H. Personality characteristics of children of alcoholics. Journal of Consulting and Clinical Psychology. 1988;**56**(2):206

[38] Sher KJ, Walitzer KS, Wood PK, Brent EE. Characteristics of children of alcoholics: Putative risk factors, substance use and abuse, and psychopathology. Journal of Abnormal Psychology. 1991;**100**(4):427-448

[39] Sher KJ, Trull TJ. Personality and disinhibitory psychopathology: alcoholism and antisocial personality disorder. Journal of Abnormal Psychology. 1994;**103**(1):92

[40] Eiden RD, Colder C, Leonard KE. The development of aggression in 18 to 48 month old children of alcoholic parents. Journal of Abnormal Child Psychology. 2006;**34**(3):393-407

[41] Eiden RD, Colder C, Edwards EP, Leonard KE. A longitudinal study of social competence among children of alcoholic and nonalcoholic parents: Role of parental psychopathology, parental warmth, and self-regulation. Psychology of Addictive Behaviors. 2009;**23**(1):36

[42] Ravaja N, Keltikangas-Järvinen K. Cloninger's temperament and character dimensions in young adulthood and their relation to characteristics of parental alcohol use and smoking. Journal of Studies on Alcohol. 2001;**62**(1):98-104

[43] Hinrichs J, DeFife J, Westen D. Personality subtypes in adolescent and adult children of alcoholics: A two part study. The Journal of Nervous and Mental Disease. 2011;**199**(7):487

[44] McGue M, Sharma A, Benson P. Parent and sibling influences on adolescent alcohol use and misuse: Evidence from a U.S. adoption cohort. Journal of Studies on Alcohol. 1996;**57**:8-18

[45] McKenna T, Pickens R. Personality characteristics of alcoholic children of alcoholics. Journal of Studies on Alcohol. 1983;**44**(4):688-700

[46] Woicik PA, Stewart SH, Pihl RO, Conrod PJ. The substance use risk profile scale: A scale measuring traits linked to reinforcement-specific substance use profiles. Addictive Behaviors. 2009;**34**(12):1042-1055

[47] Conrod PJ, Castellanos N, Mackie C. Personality-targeted interventions delay the growth of adolescent drinking and binge drinking. Journal of Child Psychology and Psychiatry. 2008;**49**(2):181-190

[48] Slutske WS, Heath AC, Madden PA, Bucholz KK, Statham DJ, Martin NG. Personality and the genetic risk for alcohol dependence. Journal of Abnormal Psychology. 2002;**111**(1):124

[49] Kim HK, Lee MH. Factors influencing resilience of adult children of alcoholics among college students. Journal of Korean Academy of Nursing. 2011;**41**(5):642-651

[50] Jennison KM, Johnson KA. Parental alcoholism as a risk factor for DSM-IV-defined alcohol abuse and dependence

in American women: The protective benefits of dyadic cohesion in marital communication. The American Journal of Drug and Alcohol Abuse. 2001;**27**(2):349-374

[51] Hinz LD. College student adult children of alcoholics: Psychological resilience or emotional distance? Journal of Substance Abuse. 1990;**2**(4):449-457

[52] Sadock B, Sadock V. Kaplan & Saddock's Synopsis of Psychiatry. Philadelphia, PA: Lippincott Williams & Wilkins; 2002

[53] Peterson Edwards E, Leonard K, Eiden R. Temperament and behavioral problems among infants in alcoholic families. Infant Mental Health Journal. 2001;**22**(3):374-392

[54] Edwards EP, Eiden RD, Leonard KE. Behavior problems in 18-to 36-month-old children of alcoholic fathers: Secure mother–infant attachment as a protective factor. Development and Psychopathology. 2006;**18**(2):395-407

[55] Díaz R, Gual A, García M, Arnau J, Pascual F, Cañuelo B, et al. Children of alcoholics in Spain: From risk to pathology. Social Psychiatry and Psychiatric Epidemiology. 2008;**43**(1):1

[56] Tarter RE, Laird SB, Kabene M, Bukstein O, Kaminer Y. Drug abuse severity in adolescents is associated with magnitude of deviation in temperament traits. British Journal of Addiction. 1990;**85**(11):1501-1504

[57] Martin CS, Earleywine M, Blackson TC, Vanyukov MM, Moss HB, Tarter RE. Aggressivity, inattention, hyperactivity, and impulsivity in boys at high and low risk for substance abuse. Journal of Abnormal Child Psychology. 1994;**22**(2):177-203

[58] Hussong AM, Wirth RJ, Edwards MC, Curran PJ, Chassin LA, Zucker RA. Externalizing symptoms among children of alcoholic parents: Entry points for an antisocial pathway to alcoholism. Journal of Abnormal Psychology. 2007;**116**(3):529

Chapter 2

# The Personality Traits as Risk Factors for the Development of Cognitive Impairment and Affective Symptomatology in Patients with COVID-19: The Pilot Study

*Vladimir V. Kalinin, Anna A. Zemlyanaya, Igor V. Damulin, Ekaterina A. Fedorenko and Maxim A. Syrtsev*

## Abstract

The current pilot study has been carried out in order to find the possible relationships between premorbid personality traits and cognitive impairments and affective symptomatology in patients recovered from COVID-19. Thirty subjects with so-called post-COVID-19 syndrome have been included into study. The diagnosis of COVID-19 has been previously confirmed by laboratory tests in each person. The control group included 30 healthy persons. For the assessment of depression and anxiety, the Hospital Anxiety and Depression Scale has been used. For the assessment of cognitive impairment, Verbal Fluency test, Montreal Cognitive Assessment (MoCA) test, and Wisconsin Card Sorting test (WCST) were used. The Munich Personality Scale and Toronto Alexithymia Scale were used for the assessment of premorbid personality. The multiple stepwise regression analysis has been used for the assessment of relationships between premorbid personality constructs and cognitive tests results and affective and anxiety symptomatology. Obtained results have shown that Frustration Tolerance test decreased the number of wrong answers in WCST and reduced the latency of the answers with positive reinforcement and also reduced the depression level and by that had the positive effects. On the other hand, Extraversion reduced the score of Montreal Cognitive Assessment (MoCA) test and increased the percentage of perseverative wrong answers in WCST-2 test and by that had negative effect on cognitive functions. Similarly, constructs of Adherence to Social Norms and Tendencies to Isolation both reduced the final MOCA score and by that predisposed to post-COVID-19 syndrome development. Esoteric tendencies construct reduced the latencies of answers with positive and negative reinforcement in WCST-3 and WCST-4 and by that had protective influence on cognitive functions. Alexithymia score correlated positively with Depression, while Neuroticism correlated positively with Anxiety.



IntechOpen

**Keywords:** personality traits, Munich Personality Test, alexithymia, post-COVID-19 syndrome, cognitive impairment, affective, anxiety symptomatology

## 1. Introduction

The COVID-19 pandemic is regarded as worldwide catastrophe that affected 225 territories and countries and lead to innumerable rate of deaths [1].

Until 2021, the confirmed case count of COVID-19 in the world surpassed over 275 million cases [1], although the real level of affected cases is thought to be much greater and 2.75 billion people may be infected by COVID-19 [2–6].

Although a great part of COVID-19-infected patients has recovered and remained alive, the serious sequels in the form of so-called post-COVID-19 syndrome have persisted.

The cognitive deficits are thought to be the frequent display of post-COVID-19 syndrome and may appear even after the milder cases of infection that have not required hospitalization [7].

A study performed by Hampshire et al. [7] has been shown that the observed deficits varied in scale with respiratory symptom severity, related to positive biological verification of having had the virus even among milder cases, could not be explained by differences in age, education, or other demographic and socioeconomic variables, remained in those who had no other residual symptoms and was of greater scale than common preexisting conditions that are associated with virus susceptibility and cognitive problems.

The deficits affected multiple tests but to different degrees. When examining the entire population, the deficits were most pronounced for paradigms that tapped cognitive functions such as reasoning, problem-solving, spatial planning, and target detection while sparing tests of simpler functions such as working-memory span as well as emotional processing. These results are in line with reports of long-COVID-19, where the so-called "brain fog" trouble concentrating and difficulty finding the correct words are common [7].

In the systematic review, performed by Rogers et al. [8], the presented data have shown that in the acute phase around third of patients experienced impaired memory, concentration, or attention, while after the illness, around one-fifth of all patients had one or more of the aforementioned cognitive impairments and about one-third of patients have experienced so-called dysexecutive syndrome consisting of "inattention, disorientation, or poorly organized movements in response to command" [8, 9].

Based on these observations, conclusion can be made that COVID-19 has the global destructive action on multiple brain functions that, in turn, can lead to impairment in quality of everyday life and loss of social adaptation [10].

In addition to cognitive deterioration, the affective symptomatology including depression and anxiety states also may be presented in the structure of post-COVID-19 syndrome [1, 6–11].

In study by Almeria et al. [11], performed on 35 patients with COVID-19, the association between neurological symptoms such as headache, loss of smell, and taste were strongly associated with impairment in several subtests including attention, memory, and executive function domains. Of the above symptoms, headache was the neurological symptom frequently associated with poor performance in *neuropsychological tests*. The authors have also showed that cognitive impairment was found in patients who required oxygen therapy during hospitalization. They explained it by the continuous hypoxia caused by pulmonary disease related to COVID-19 infection. Headache and oxygen therapy independently were the main variables strongly related to cognitive impairment. In patients with these symptoms, global Cognitive Index was impaired. Patients presenting diarrhea during infection had worse performance in neuropsychological test [11].

Although the numerous clinical data confirmed the role of severe somatic symptomatology in the genesis neurocognitive deficit in COVID-19 patients [6–11], the role of premorbid personality constructs for the development of cognitive impairment and concomitant affective pathology remains unknown. Obviously, that if such relationship really exists, it may prepare the physicians in advance to more intensive and specific approach to treatment of such patients. In other words, the investigations on the relationships between premorbid personality constructs and post-COVID-19 syndrome are utterly required.

The studies of relationships between premorbid personality types and following depression development have a long history in modern psychiatry. Many authors since antiquity tried to find the connections between them. In this context, the studies of Abraham concerning the so-called oral structure of character, Kretschmer's Cycloid personality, and Shimoda's description of so-called Statothymia should be mentioned [12].

The work of Tellenbach presenting the so-called Typus Melancholicus (TM) has also regarded that personality construct as risk factor for the following monopolar depression development [13]. According to this model, such traits as orderliness, conscientiousness, hyper/hetereonomia, and intolerance of ambiguity are the core features of Typus Melancholicus (TM). Previous studies showed a relationship between unipolar depression and TM construct [12–14].

Moreover, the new formalized scales for the assessment of premorbid personality traits, such as Munich personality scale [15] and Toronto Alexithymia scale [16], were elaborated, and question about their capability for the assessment of premorbid personality structure for the prediction of following depression development has not been yet resolved.

Here also should emphasize that modern psychometric formalized scales have not been yet used for study on relationships between premorbid personality on the one hand and affective symptomatology and cognitive deterioration on the other hand in post-COVID-19 syndrome.

## 2. Objective

The current pilot study has been designed and performed in order to find the possible relationships between premorbid personality traits and cognitive impairments and affective symptomatology in patients recovered from COVID-19 in persons with post-COVID-19 syndrome.

## 3. Material and methods

For the current study, 30 subjects with so-called post-COVID-19 syndrome have been selected and included into study. All patients had neither chronic somatic nor mental illnesses. Among studied persons were 11 males and 19 females. The mean age of studied patient was 30.8 + −14.5 and varied from 19 to 64 years.

The diagnosis of COVID-19 has been previously confirmed by laboratory tests in each person. The mean duration of time since recovery was 1.78 + −0.9 and varied from 1 to 4 months.

For the comparison purposes, the control group of healthy persons has been formed. It included 30 healthy persons, who have not been infected by COVID-19, and it was confirmed by negative results in COVID-19 tests. The control group included 10 males and 20 females. The mean age of control group was 28.9 + −12.7 and varied from 18 to 62 years. There was no statistically significant discrepancy in age between groups.

For the assessment of depression and anxiety, all patients were evaluated by psychiatrists in order to assess the affective and cognitive state. For these purposes, the Hospital Anxiety and Depression Scale has been used [17].

For the assessment of cognitive traits, the Montreal Cognitive Assessment (MoCA-test) [18, 19], Wisconsin card sorting test (WCST), [20] and Verbal Fluency test [21, 22] were used.

For the assessment of the premorbid personality features, the Munich Personality Test (MPT) has been used [14].

The MPT represents a self-rating questionnaire and includes 51 questions depicting the different personality traits. The patients have filled in all rating scales themselves, and after that the obtained raw data have been transformed into six constructs in line with specific structure of scales. These constructs include Extraversion, Neuroticism, Rigidity, Frustration Tolerance, Tendencies to Isolation, and Esoteric Tendency. The last two constructs form Schizoidia scale [12]. The other two control scales of MPT (Orientation toward Social Norms and Motivation) were not included in the final analysis.

Extraversion and Neuroticism constructs are derived from Eysenck and Eysenck concepts [23]. Rigidity is quite similar to construct of Typus Melancholicus proposed by Tellenbach [12, 13], while Tendency to Isolation and Esoteric Tendency are based on Kretschmer's classical study on relationships between constitution and personality [14]. Frustration Tolerance refers to resiliency or stress coping strategy.

Along with MPT, the Toronto Alexithymia Scale (TAS-26) [24] was explored for the assessment of alexithymia. The choice of alexithymia scale was explained by the facts that alexithymia itself is often connected with other disorders, such as post-traumatic stress disorder (PTSD) and Holocaust survivors [15, 16].

TAS-26 consists of 26 items, and each item can be scored in points from 1 to 5. The global alexithymia score in TAS-26 may be expressed from 26 to 130 points [24]. All patients with global TAS-26 score who exceed 74 points were regarded as persons with alexithymia. The values of TAS-26 varied from 40.00 to 75.00, and mean value in post-COVID-19 syndrome achieved 58.27 + − 9.69.

## 4. Statistical analysis

The multiple regression analysis has been used in order to find any possible relationships between premorbid personality traits on the one hand and affective symptomatology and variables of cognitive impairments in COVID-19 patients on the other hand [25, 26].

In the control group, such analysis of relationship between premorbid personality and clinical manifestation has not been performed, since the primary aim of the current pilot study was research of mentioned above correlations in COVID-19 patients but not in healthy persons.

## 5. Results

The main obtained results are shown in the next tables. In **Table 1**, the comparison of means of cognitive variables and affective syndromes between post-COVID-19 syndrome patients and healthy control subjects are presented.

As can be seen between the patients with post-COVID-19 syndrome and healthy control persons, a great statistically significant difference exists. It concerns used test on cognitive functions and implies the severe mental cognitive deterioration due the transitory COVID-19 infection. Similarly, the level of depression and anxiety states was higher in post-COVID-19 patients.

**Table 2** shows the results of multiple regression analysis for the relationships between the main premorbid personality traits and cognitive variables in post-COVID-19 syndrome patients.

As can be seen, only two personality traits had no influence on cognitive tests. They included TAS-26 and Neuroticism (MPT). The other four premorbid personality constructs had statistically significant influence on five cognitive tests except the VFT.

Thus, there was a statistically significant negative association between Frustration Tolerance and the level of the percentage of wrong answers, the representation of perseverative wrong answers, and the latency of the answers with positive reinforcement, i.e. this personality construct had the positive and protective influence on WCST performance in post-COVID-19 syndrome.

On the other hand, Extraversion construct reduced the score of MOCA test and increased the percentage of perseverative wrong answers in WCST-2 test that implies

| Variable | Post-COVID-19 syndrome patients (n = 30) | Healthy control persons (n = 30) | Significance |
|---|---|---|---|
| Verbal Fluency test (VFT) | 12.68 + −4.47 | 16.80 + −2.14 | p = 0.0000 |
| MOCA test | 26.55 + −1.90 | 27.80 + −1.15 | p = 0.0031 |
| WCST-1 | 27.95 + −14.54 | 18.50 + −3.0 | p = 0.0009 |
| WCST-2 | 15.27 + −7.24 | 9.1 + −1.85 | p = 0.0000 |
| WCST-3 | 2.99 + −1.35 | 1.72 + −0.63 | p = 0.0000 |
| WCST-4 | 4.53 + −2.21 | 2.62 + −1.32 | p = 0.0001 |
| Depression (HADS) | 5.55 + − 4.13 | 2.63 + −1.60 | p = 0.0006 |
| Anxiety (HADS) | 5.82 + −4.75 | 2.80 + −1.35 | p = 0.0014 |

**Note:** *all statistically significant values of beta coefficients and R2 are marked in boldface.*
*MOCA – Montreal cognitive assessment; WCST-1 – the percentage of wrong answers; WCST-2 – the percentage of perseverative wrong answers; WCST-3 – the latency of answers with positive reinforcement in seconds; WCST-4 – the latency of answers with negative reinforcement in seconds.*

**Table 1.**
*Comparison of mean values of different cognitive tests values and depression and anxiety in post-COVID-19 patients and health normal control persons.*

| Variable | Verbal Fluency (VFT) | MOCA | WCST-1 | WCST-2 | WCST-3 | WCST-4 |
|---|---|---|---|---|---|---|
| Beta TAS-26 | — | — | — | — | — | — |
| Beta Frustration Tolerance | — | — | **−0.572** | **−0.811** | **−0.630** | — |
| Beta Neuroticism | — | — | — | — | — | — |
| Beta Extraversion | — | **−0.675** | — | **0.573** | — | — |
| Beta Social norms | — | **−0.725** | — | — | — | — |
| Beta Isolation tendencies | — | **−0.527** | — | — | — | — |
| Beta Esoteric tendencies | — | — | — | — | **−0.441** | **−0.528** |
| R2 (Explained total variance) | - | **0.599** | **0.327** | **0.513** | **0.591** | **0.279** |

*Note: all statistically significant values of beta coefficients and R2 are marked in boldface.*
**MOCA** – *Montreal cognitive assessment;* **WCST-1** – *the percentage of wrong answers;* **WCST-2** – *the percentage of perseverative wrong answers;* **WCST-3** – *the latency of answers with positive reinforcement in seconds;* **WCST-4** – *the latency of answers with negative reinforcement in seconds.*

**Table 2.**
*Multiple regression analysis (values of beta coefficients) for some cognitive tests as dependent variable on different premorbid personality states.*

the destructive effect of that construct on cognitive functions in COVID-19-infected patients.

Similarly, the personality constructs of Adherence to Social Norms and Tendencies to Isolation both reduced the final MOCA score and by that had destructive influence on cognitive functions in post-COVID-19 syndrome patients.

Quite the contrary, the Esoteric Tendencies construct reduced the latencies of answers with positive and negative reinforcement in WCST-3 and WCST-4 and by that had positive influence on cognitive performance in COVID-19 patients.

Concerning the mentioned results, should be also stressed that the maximal value of explained variance ($R2 = 0.591$) has been revealed for WCST-3. IT implies that Frustration Tolerance and Esoteric Tendencies constructs are maximally effective in the prediction of WCST-3.

Analysis of relationships between premorbid personality traits and affective symptomatology in post-COVID-19 syndrome patients (See **Table 3**) revealed that Frustration Tolerance correlated negative ($\beta = -0.465$) with Depression and by that exerted protective influence on Depression development, while the Alexithymia score correlated positively with Depression and by that determined the higher Depression score.

On the other hand, the Neuroticism construct correlated positively ($\beta = 0.737$) with Anxiety score that implies the anxiety symptomatology increase in patients with high Neuroticism level.

| Variable | Depression (HADS) | Anxiety (HADS) |
|---|---|---|
| Beta TAS-26 | **0.577** | — |
| Beta<br>Frustration Tolerance | **-0.465** | — |
| Beta<br>Neuroticism | — | **0.737** |
| Beta<br>Extraversion | — | — |
| Beta<br>Social norms | — | — |
| Beta<br>Isolation tendencies | — | — |
| Beta<br>Esoteric Tendencies | — | — |
| R2<br>(Explained total variance) | **0.719** | **0.543** |

*Note: all statistically significant values of beta coefficients and R2 are marked in bold.*

**Table 3.**
*Multiple regression analysis (values of beta coefficients) for affective constructs on different premorbid personality states.*

## 6. Discussion

Personality traits are thought to be important characteristics, since they may predispose to the development of some psychopathological condition, including affective and anxiety states [12–16]. The main problem in this context concerns the probability of concrete psychopathological state prediction based on the basis of premorbid personality traits before the mental disorder development.

Moreover, the definite answer to the question whether the personality traits can predispose or not to affective disorder after the influence of any exogenous factors (such as COVID-19) is absent.

Similarly, there is also absent the definite answer to the question on the relationships between premorbid personality structure and subsequent development of cognitive impairment after COVID-19 infection [8–11].

The current pilot study has been designed and performed in order to respond to all these posed questions.

The study may be criticized for the small number of selected patients. In order to overcome such shortcoming, the meticulous statistical method in form of regression analysis was used.

The main results of the current study have shown that persons who suffered by COVID-19 infection really are characterized by some neurocognitive impairments including Verbal Fluency, MOCA tests, and Wisconsin Card Sorting Test.

Moreover, the premorbid personality was really connected with some cognitive tests and subsequent affective and anxiety syndromes development.

Principally that different premorbid personality constructs influenced wide-ranging upon cognitive functions. Thus, Extraversion, Adherence to Social Norms, and Tendencies to Isolation reduced the MOCA score and by that disturbed the cognitive functions. While, Frustration Tolerance reduced the number of wrong answers and perseverative wrong answers and by that improved the final results in WCST.

Similarly, Frustration Tolerance reduced the latency of answering with positive reinforcement, while Esoteric Tendencies reduced the latencies as with positive, as with negative reinforcement and by that both these personality constructs again improved cognitive functions.

Utterly in line with these results are the findings on the negative correlation between Frustration Tolerance and Depression development in post-COVID-19 syndrome. Here, the positive correlation between Frustration Tolerance and Depression also should be mentioned. Principally, that combination of Alexithymia state and Frustration Tolerance lead to maximal explained variance of Depression score, i.e. the combination of these two constructs may predict the Depression appearance more precisely than any other factors.

Principally, that Rigidity construct that corresponds to "Typus Melancholicus" in studies by Tellenbach [12–14] had no statistically significant relationships with Depression. The cause of such contradiction remains unknown and probably may be explained by pathogenetic differences in endogenous depression and depression in post-COVID-19 syndrome.

The current study can also be criticized for the lack of similar statistical analysis in the control group. Nevertheless, it was not done since the primary aim of the current study concerned the search of relationships between premorbid personality constructs and cognitive impairment and affective symptomatology in patients suffering from COVID-19 and not in control health persons.

An analysis of relationships between premorbid personality constructs and cognitive impairment and psychopathology in the control healthy group was beyond the present study and has not been performed, since the healthy persons have no any severe symptomatology. It may be done in the special work in the nearest future.

Conclusion can be made that the low score of Frustration Tolerance and Esoteric Tendencies has unfavorable influence on cognitive functions in patients with post-COVID-19 syndrome, while the high scores of these constructs cause the protective effect against cognitive deterioration and Depression development.

## Author details

Vladimir V. Kalinin*, Anna A. Zemlyanaya, Igor V. Damulin, Ekaterina A. Fedorenko and Maxim A. Syrtsev
Department of Organic Brain Disorders and Epilepsy, Moscow Research Institute of Psychiatry - The Branch of Serbsky's National Center of Psychiatry and Narcology, Ministry of Health of Russian Federation, Moscow, Russian Federation

*Address all correspondence to: doct.kalinin@mail.ru

## References

[1] Ceban F, Susan LS, Lu ILMW, Lee Y, Gill H, Teopiz KM, et al. Fatigue and cognitive impairment in Post-COVID-19 syndrome: A systematic review and meta-analysis. Brain, Behavior and Immunity. 2022;**101**:93-135

[2] Wu SL, Mertens AN, Crider YS, Nguyen A, Pokpongkiat NN, Djajadi S, et al. Substantial underestimation of SARS-CoV-2 infection in the United States. Nature Communications. 2020;**11**(1)

[3] Havers FP, Reed C, Lim T, Montgomery JM, Klena JD, Hall AJ, et al. Seroprevalence of antibodies to SARS-CoV-2 in 10 sites in the United States. JAMA Internal Medicine. 2020;**180**(12):1576

[4] Aizenman N. Why the pandemic is 10 times worse than you think. NPR. Available from: https://www.npr.org/sections/health-shots/2021/02/06/964527835/why-the-pandemic-is-10-times-worse-than-you-think. Published February 6, 2021. Accessed May 19, 2021

[5] Huang C, Huang L, Wang Y, Li X, Ren L, Gu X, et al. 6-month consequences of COVID-19 in patients discharged from hospital: A cohort study. Lancet. 2021;**397**(10270):220-232

[6] Renaud-Charest O, Lui LMW, Eskander S, Ceban F, Ho R, Di Vincenzo JD, et al. Onset and frequency of depression in post-COVID-19 syndrome: A systematic review. Journal of Psychiatric Research. 2021;**144**:129-137

[7] Hampshire A, Trender W, Chamberlain SR, Jolly AE, Grant JE, Patrick F, et al. Cognitive deficits in people who have recovered from COVID-19. EClinical Medicine. 2021;**39**:101044

[8] Rogers JP, Chesney E, Oliver D, Pollak TA, McGuire P, Fusar-Poli P, et al. Psychiatric and neuropsychiatric presentations associated with severe coronavirus infections: A systematic review and meta-analysis with comparison to the COVID-19 pandemic. Lancet Psychiatry. 2020;**7**:611-627. DOI: 10.1016/S2215-0366(20)30203-0

[9] Daroische R, Hemminghyth MS, Eilertsen TH, Breitve MH, Chwiszczuk LJ. Cognitive impairment after COVID-19-a review on objective test data. Frontiers in Neurology. 2021;**12**:699582. DOI: 10.3389/FNEUR.2021.699582

[10] Atuna M, Sanchez-Saudinos MB, Lleo A. Cognitive symptoms after COVID-19. Neurology Perspectives. 2021;**1**:S16-S24

[11] Almeria M, Cejudo JC, Sotoca J, Deus J, Krupinski J. Cognitive profile following COVID-19 infection: Clinical predictors leading to neuropsychological impairment. Brain, Behavior & Immunity-Health. 2020;**9**:100163

[12] Marneros A. Das neue Handbuch der Bipolaren und Depressiven Erkrankungen, Georg Thieme Verlag, Stuttgart. 2004. p. 781

[13] Tellenbach H. Melancholie. Problemgeschichte, Endogenitat, Typologie, Pathogenese, Klinik. Heidelberg, New York, Berlin: Springer Verlag; 1961. p. 280

[14] Zerssen D, von Pfister H, Koeller D-M. The munich personality test (MPT): A short questionnaire for

self-rating and relatives' rating of personality traits: Formal properties and clinical potential. European Archives of Psychiatry and Neurological Sciences. 1988;**238**:73-93

[15] Shipko S, Alvarez WA, Noviello N. Towards a teleological model of alexithymia: Alexithymia and post-traumatic stress disorder. Psychotherapy and Psychosomatics. 1983;**39**(2):122-126. DOI: 10.1159/000287730

[16] Yehuda R, Steiner A, Kahana B, Binder-Brynes K, Southwick SM, Zemelman S, et al. Alexithymia in Holocaust survivors with and without PTSD. Journal of Traumatic Stress. 1997;**10**(1):83-100. DOI: 10.1002/

[17] Zigmond AS, Snaith RP. The hospital anxiety and depression scale. Acta Psychiatrica Scandinavica. 1983;**67**(6):361-370

[18] Nasreddine ZS, Phillips NA, Bédirian V, Charbonneau S, Whitehead V, Collin I, et al. The Montreal cognitive assessment, MoCA: A brief screening tool for mild cognitive impairment. Journal of the American Geriatrics Society. 2005;**53**(4):695-999

[19] Borland E, Nägga K, Nilsson PM, Minthon L, Nilsson ED, Palmqvist S. The Montreal cognitive assessment: Normative data from a large swedish population-based cohort. Journal of Alzheimer's Disease. 2017;**59**(3):893-901

[20] Monchi O, Petrides M, Petre V, Worsley K, Dagher A. Wisconsin card sorting revisited: Distinct neural circuits participating in different stages of the task identified by event-related functional magnetic resonance imaging. The Journal of Neuroscience. 2001;**21**(19):7733-7741

[21] Borkowski JG, Benton AL, Spreen O. Word fluency and brain damage. Neuropsychologia. 1967;**5**(2):135-140

[22] Ross T. The reliability of cluster and switch scores for the controlled oral word association test. Archives of Clinical Neuropsychology. 2003;**18**(2):153-164

[23] Eysenck HJ, Eysenck SBG. Manual of the Eysenck Personality Inventory. London: Hodder & Stoughton; 1975

[24] Bagby RM, Taylor GJ, Ryan D. Toronto alexithymia scale: Relationship with personality and psychopathology measures. Psychotherapy and Psychosomatics. 1986;**45**:207-215

[25] Feinstein AR. Principles of Medical Statistics. Boca Raton: Chapman & Hall/CDS; 2002. p. 701

[26] Mathews DE, Farewell VT. Using and Understanding Medical Statistics. Basel: Karger; 2007. p. 322

Section 2

# The Psychopathology of Neuropsychiatric Disorders

**Chapter 3**

# Individual Education Support System Using ICT for Developmental Disabilities

*Sakiko Ogoshi, Yasuhiro Ogoshi, Tohru Saitoh, Kotoko Tanaka, Yoichi Itoh, Masahiro Wakamatu, Tomoyuki Kanno and Akio Nakai*

## Abstract

Children with developmental disabilities require special support to help them in different aspects of daily life, and individual educational support is a crucial part of such support. We developed a collaborative system for supporting children with developmental disabilities using ICT to be used by teachers, parents, and supporters. This chapter introduces this system, which provides close and immediate support through instantaneously sharing daily behavior information about the child between teacher-parent-supporters. In addition, storing the data in a highly secure cloud system facilitates passing information to children's next educational level. Moreover, AI can match support needs and support services according to the characteristics of individual children by using ICF codes for suggesting immediate, dynamic support.

**Keywords:** individual education support system, ICT, developmental disabilities, assistive technology, educational technology

## 1. Introduction

A survey conducted in Japan by the Ministry of Education, Culture, Sports, Science, and Technology targeting children with ADHD [1], ASD [2, 3], LD [4], SLD, and DCD [5, 6] characteristics revealed that approximately 6.3% of children need support. Therefore, the Ministry advocated promoting special support education. In 2003, the Ministry's "Future of Special Support Education (Final Report)" proposed the creation of "Individualized Educational Support Plans" as one mechanism for responding to the diverse needs of young children with disabilities appropriately. As a result, the "Individualized Educational Support Plan" and "Individualized Guidance Plan" were included in study courses.

Subsequently, in 2004, the Law for Supporting Persons with Developmental Disabilities was enacted, which legally defined developmental disabilities for the first time in Japan. Its basic principles also state that "support shall be provided to persons with developmental disabilities according to their age, sex, the disability status, individual living conditions, and the needs of related government and private sector organizations, engaged in medical, health, welfare, education, labor, and other associated services." Support programs must be conducted seamlessly in close coordination with other organizations while supporting the decision-making process.

However, neither the creation of "individualized educational support plans" nor "individualized instructional plans" nor appropriate education and support based on these plans have been widely implemented in actual educational settings. In response to this situation, the 2016 revision of the Act on Support for Persons with Developmental Disabilities Article 8 stipulates "the preparation of individualized educational support plans, i.e., plans regarding individualized long-term support conducted in collaboration with relevant organizations engaged in work related to education, and relevant organizations and private organizations engaged in work related to medical care, health, welfare, and labor, among others," which refers to the preparation of a report on the status of company business. The Government of Japan shall take other necessary measures, such as promoting the preparation of plans for bullying prevention and individual guidance, promoting measures to prevent bullying, and developing other support systems. The new law includes the following provisions. Furthermore, the Ministry of Education, Culture, Sports, Science and Technology's "Courses of Study for Special Needs Schools (2017)" states cooperation between school and the home. "In consideration of the child or student's developmental stage, the child or student, the language activities of the child or student shall be enriched, and consideration shall be given to helping the child or student establish study habits in cooperation with the home."

The report "Promoting Special Support Education for the Establishment of an Inclusive Education System Toward the Formation of a Coexisting Society (Subcommittee on Elementary and Secondary Education, Central Council for Education, 2012)" states the following about cooperation and support with parents, "Close cooperation between school and home is important in providing support for children with disabilities. For example, the school where the child with disabilities is enrolled and the home should regularly share information about the child's progress and clarify the roles of each." In 2018, the Triangle Project, which is a cooperative project between families, education, and welfare, was designed to provide parents, guardians, and medical institutions measures to "promote further cooperation between families, education, and welfare so that children with disabilities and their parents/guardians can receive seamless support in the community" [7]. In response to the report, the Ministerial Ordinance partially revised the Enforcement Regulations of the School Education Law.

"When a school prepares an individualized educational support plan," the school shall prepare it in cooperation with relevant organizations and private organizations such as medical, welfare, health, and labor, among others (after this, referred to as "relevant organizations, among others."), while taking into consideration the wishes of the students concerned or their guardians. Moreover, in preparing an individual educational support plan for a school, the school shall share necessary information regarding support for said students, among others, with relevant medical, welfare, health, labor, and other organizations and private organizations (after this referred to as "relevant organizations, among others."), while considering the wishes of said students, among others, and their guardians. In addition, regarding handover, "it is essential to provide consistent support for students with disabilities from early childhood to after graduation from school from a long-term perspective, including school life and life at home and the community." Therefore, schools should prepare an individualized educational support plan that includes the individuals and their guardians. The significance of transitions was also included, "After obtaining the consent of the students, the school should pass appropriate information about them to their next schools of higher education, among others."

As mentioned above, school teachers need to create individual educational support plans and individual guidance plans for children with developmental disabilities in cooperation with their families and community supporters, and provide consistent support over a long period of time; however, it is currently difficult to do so sufficiently because teachers are too busy. Therefore, the current situation of developmental disabilities in Japan and the current state of the educational field (online, basic information as a subject) call for familiar, prompt, and effective support through the accumulation of daily activity histories using ICT. As described below, the use of ICT in education is progressing, and in Fukui Prefecture, tablet terminals have been distributed to all students and the ICT environment is being developed.

Therefore, the primary objectives of this study are 1) to establish a system that allows schools, parents, and support organizations to share information on children's behavior immediately and dynamically, leading to smooth support; and 2) to establish a system that allows schools, parents, and support organizations to share information on children's behavior immediately and dynamically, leading to smooth support. For this purpose, a cloud system was considered necessary and developed. Furthermore, 2) the second objective is to provide support devices that meet the individual characteristics of people with developmental disabilities. To achieve these two objectives, we developed a system using ICT technology, which can be used jointly by schools, families, and support organizations to solve problems.

Section 3 describes the system configuration, and Section 4 describes feedback to the support plan and progress for further development based on the configuration. Section 4 introduces the support devices and services developed based on the needs of supporters of children with developmental disabilities. Section 5 provides a summary of the discussion.

## 2. Educational support using ICT

The GIGA school concept in contemporary Japan promotes the development of a one-on-one terminal per student environment. In Fukui Prefecture, tablet terminals have been installed for all students. Highly advanced ICT education will be introduced to educational practices conducted to date. This innovation in education is expected to contribute to fair and individualized learning that leaves no one behind and fosters creativity in diverse children, significantly expands possibilities for children with special needs, and increases the options for supporting children with developmental disabilities. In Japan, teachers are faced with a large workload, and accelerating the introduction and operation of ICT, including integrated school administration support systems, will help reduce class preparation and grade processing burdens. It is also hoped that ICT would lead to a reform of schools' working styles. We must not forget that the development of an ICT environment is a means and not an end. It is being undertaken to ensure that children are equipped with abundant creativity and develop the necessary qualities and abilities to live independently in the unpredictable future and participate in developing society as creators of a sustainable society. It is critical to nurture children's ability to use information, including Internet literacy, to use ICT appropriately and safely.

Prior studies have reported case studies on online classes and online diagnostics [8, 9]. In previous studies, there have been numerous research and development efforts on devices and services to support children with developmental disabilities [10]. However, there is no other system that shares information on daily student behavior between school, family, and specialized agencies and matches it with appropriate support devices and services.

This section introduces a system undergoing research and development in Fukui Prefecture since 2009 to support children with developmental disabilities using ICT. The system connects schools, families, and specialized institutions and provides support while sharing daily information about children with homeroom teachers, guardians, and supporters.

## 3. Individualized education support system using ICT to link schools, families, and specialized institutions

### 3.1 Development of a collaborative support system according to individual characteristics

Before talking about systems, we would like to discuss some critical points about providing support. It is often said that supporting developmentally disabled children is very difficult. One reason is that the condition of a child with developmental disabilities often changes over time. Sometimes they are in good shape, and sometimes in bad shape. It is difficult to understand the child's condition because every child is different. It is easy to assume that support, which worked well for one child, would also work for another child. Often, identical support does not work for different children. In addition, in many cases, children are good at what they do. As a result, people around children tend to think that children can do these things. Therefore, if children cannot do what is expected, people think they fail on purpose or are not authentic. In addition, children with developmental disabilities might not be able to repeat what they do well in one place in another place.

Moreover, it is difficult for individuals to understand their failures. These characteristics demand early recognition and support that matches individual needs. Early detection and observations are critical for supporting children with developmental disabilities. Each person feels and learns differently during parenting. Therefore, it is necessary to understand and recognize the characteristics and differences of each child when providing education suitable for their characteristics.

It is critical to observe each person, regardless of their disability; therefore, it is necessary to keep the child closely and precisely. Furthermore, it is required to do this on an uninterrupted and continuous basis in close cooperation with the school, family, and specialists. In addition, close collaboration is essential for a supportive environment. It is often stated that successful people with developmental disabilities always have a supportive key person. In the case of children, the key person is usually the homeroom teacher, parents, club or cram school teachers, or other supporters. For example, if the homeroom teacher and parents do their best to support the child but do so in opposite directions, they might become confused and unsure of what is best for them. Therefore, it is also necessary to have a common understanding between homeroom teachers and parents through close cooperation and collaboration. In addition, if a child continues to make mistakes, their environment might become cold in terms of human relations. Therefore, it is necessary to create a place where adults can support the child and help the child experience success in maintaining the warmth of the surroundings.

It is now mandatory to develop Individualized Educational Support Plans; however, transitional support, which is handing over a child's history to the next level, is rarely adequate. Parents are especially burdened by the frequency of completing and submitting their child's history to different agencies providing support. Teachers are also burdened by the large amount of paperwork related to special needs, including the Individualized Educational Support Plan. When a child moves to the next grade or higher education, there is an increasing risk of losing an opportunity to learn if too much time is spent understanding a child's characteristics. Therefore, transferring the child's history and ongoing support is essential [11]. Childhood is an exercise in developing the ability to live. Therefore, failures are necessary experiences. It is necessary to give children the opportunity to succeed when they make a mistake. It is also essential to gradually develop their ability to live by turning experiences of failure in elementary schools into successful experiences in junior high schools, technical colleges, high schools, and universities, and gradually connect these successful experiences to the real world of employment and employment continuity. The continuous transfer of information plays a vital role in achieving this goal. Therefore, a system for recording information about daily activities in close chronological order is necessary for understanding the conditions and behaviors of each individual and sharing this information continuously with support providers. In addition, busy teachers, supporters, and parents have less time today due to their busy schedules. Therefore, it might be impossible to provide 100% support for children with developmental disabilities in this busy and information-overloaded age, regardless of the enthusiasm and talents of teachers, parents, and professionals. As a result, a system is needed to collect information to understand children's characteristics for providing support according to individual needs. A system is also required for sharing daily information quickly among all parties involved. In addition, supporting many children with developmental disabilities is one of watching and waiting because the type of support that should be provided is unclear even after the child's characteristics are identified.

As a result, a system that dynamically and immediately matches individuals with support resources, including people, equipment, the environment, and individual characteristics, is needed. Therefore, we developed a system to solve the above issues consisting of a web cloud platform system and assistive AI to support people by providing individualized educational support through the collaboration between people and AI. We are currently conducting a new experiment with the cooperation of the Fukui Prefectural Teachers Association and elementary, junior high, and special-needs schools in Fukui Prefecture to demonstrate the system. The individualized Education Support System in Fukui Prefecture was developed by developmental disabilities specialists, parents' associations of children with developmental disabilities, and the teachers. The system's operation was established with the cooperation of Fukui Prefecture's elementary and junior high special-needs schools and teachers' unions. We developed the first version of an "ICT system called Picotto for connecting parents, schools, developmental disabilities specialists and their supporters." Beginning in 2009, we operated the system and conducted demonstration tests. Strong security and personal information management are required for managing and using this platform. Therefore, Hitachi Solutions East Japan, Ltd. was contracted to manage and operate the system from 2021. **Figure 1a** shows a use case of the system. **Figure 1b** shows a diagram of the systems' overview.

As seen in **Figure 1**, the system allows parents, homeroom teachers, and supporters involved with each student to set up checkpoints for each child based on their characteristics and goals and check these checkpoints daily and write comments. The

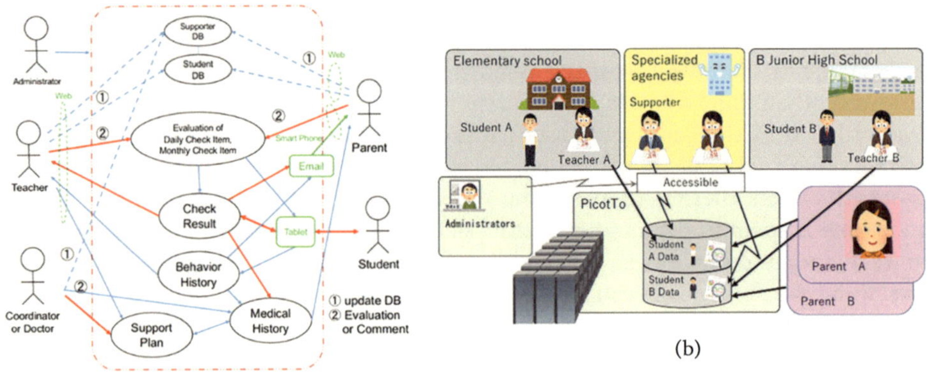

(a) (b)

**Figure 1.**
*(a) Use case of the system (b) diagram of the systems' overview.*

homeroom teachers at school also check five items related to each child daily and write comments. Also, parents or guardians check approximately five items for each child at home and write comments. The checklist consists of items corresponding to the individual's educational support and instructional plan goals. If a support person is present, they can also include information. Information sharing about behavior checks and comments using the system is immediate and stored in a database. It analyzes and visualizes this data, which will be explained in detail later. It also suggests and displays assistive devices and support services. Each behavior check item is tied to the relevant code in ICF-CY [12] inside the system. Support devices and support services are also registered by tying them to the relevant codes in ICF-CY. Therefore, AI can derive necessary support services by performing operations based on taking the product of the behavior history and the ICF-CY codes of support devices and services and adding them together. However, case study meetings are also held to include experts' opinions, and if necessary, support devices and support materials can be developed. Teaching materials and support services are not limited to academic subjects but include information on food, clothing, shelter, and social skills, considered educational. New interventions such as supportive devices are added to the daily routine in response to this feedback, and this spiral is continued by providing support and developing a child's history.

Teachers and parents conducting simple checks of these items on a PC or a tablet can accumulate daily information about the child at school and home. The system allows information sharing between the student, the family, and specialized institutions. Such information sharing facilitates understanding of students' conditions' medium- and long-term progress, enabling the chronological management of children's growth and developmental process. An example of such a screen is shown in **Figure 2**.

**Figure 2** shown here was entered by a homeroom teacher having a student with a sleep disorder. The screen contains items such as "Greetings given" and "Did not sleep during class." Moreover, there is a space on one side of the screen to write additional explanations about the checked items (**Video 1**: https://youtu.be/h8ekbDrvqhY). In addition, based on the values of items that are checked daily, evaluation points are assigned to items on learning, physical, language, interpersonal, daily living, and emotions. They are presented in an easy-to-understand radar chart format (**Figure 3**).

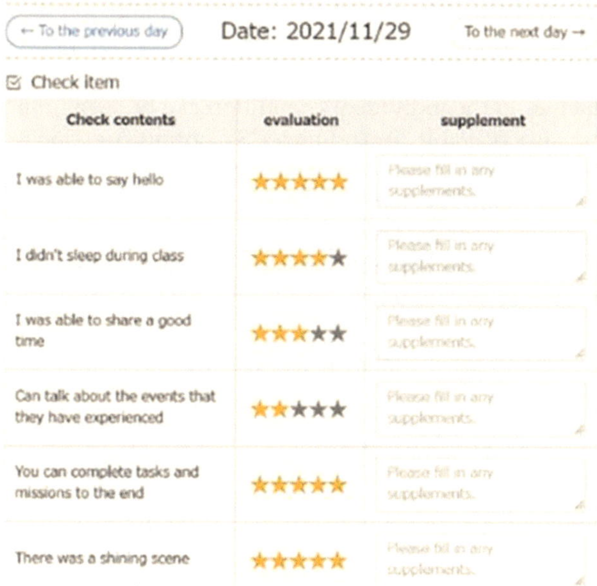


**Figure 2.**
*A screen for conducting daily checks.*

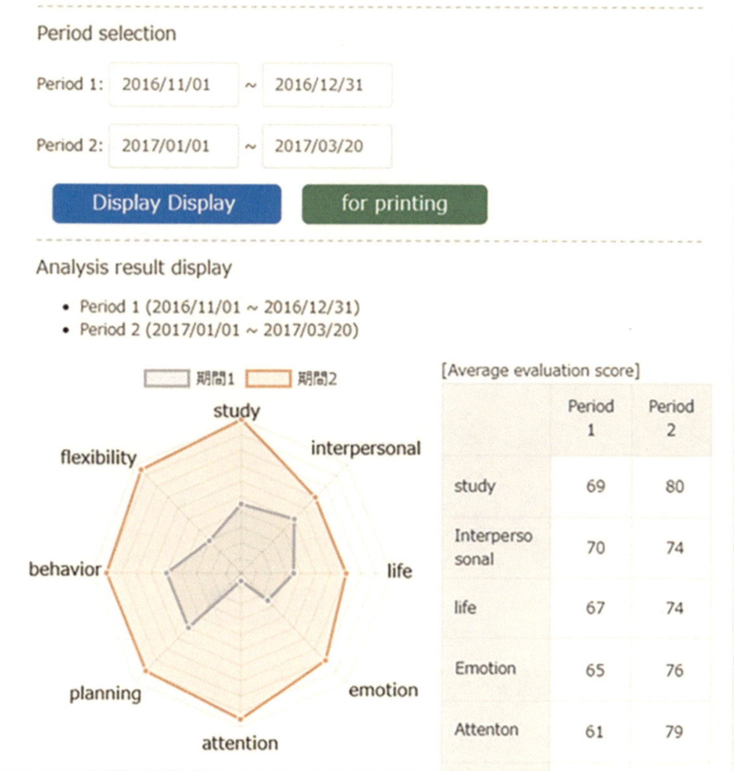


**Figure 3.**
*Visualization of behavioral changes using radar graphs.*

In this display format, the difference between the maximum and minimum values is visualized as maximum. It is also possible to display evaluation points. The current system version facilitates selecting two periods and displaying two patterns simultaneously so that changes in the individual's condition can be seen immediately. Various other interfaces are also available, including a CSV output function.

In this PoC (Proof of Concept), we have designed and developed support devices when necessary according to the status picture of the individual. The IoT (Internet of Things) support devices we have developed provide support while automatically collecting data on the student's behavior, and we have added functions that enable a detailed understanding of the student's condition and reduce the burden on teachers and parents.

We will briefly explain the mechanism for collecting action data from this IoT support device.

This system has an API (Application Programming Interface) designed to allow the addition of behavioral data and comments from various external assistive devices and educational materials.

Information from outside sources can also be stored in the device (**Figure 4**), allowing easy integration with external services.

The evaluation from the externally linked supporting devices is set as behavior check item, and the five levels of assessments are stored in the daily behavior history of students, similar to school teachers' and guardians' daily evaluations. This figure shows a screenshot of a day's history. You can see the evaluations entered by school teachers, parents, students, and the day-to-day behavior evaluations automatically accumulated by the device.

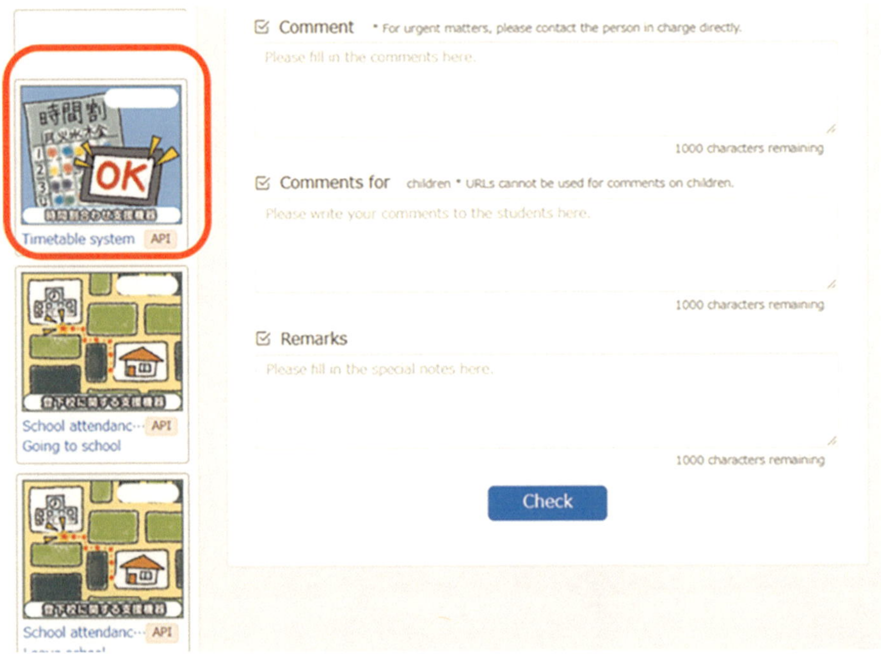


**Figure 4.**
*The user can select action items in this system when the "External linkage" checkbox is checked on the external linkage function screen.*

Next, we will explain how these assistive devices and support services are matched with individual characteristics. Picotto performs daily behavioral checks, and each behavioral item is weighted and tied to a related ICF code. Different support devices and support services are also associated with ICF codes related to the cognitive functions they support. For example, ICF code d710 is related to basic interpersonal interactions. Therefore, assessment and support tools for interpersonal relationships related to fundamental interpersonal interactions, such as situational awareness training support systems, would be identified by this ICF code.

Thus, behavioral checks by teachers, parents, supporters, and assistive devices can be collected, and data regarding the individual's strengths and weaknesses can be analyzed using this system. Furthermore, we have developed a function that expresses daily items using ICF codes, which matches and introduces support devices, teaching materials, and support services. This function enables matching students with external support services without exposing their personal information. Thus, system can immediately provide support services according to the individual characteristics and the current condition of a child. If you need to see more information, you can press "See More" to display additional information. Using this system, teachers and parents can conduct daily checks and identify support suggestions through ICF collaboration according to the characteristics of individual children.

This is the management screen of the system. Currently, it has 1500 behavior items already incorporated, and these behavior items are tied to ICF codes and weighted. ICF codes are also assigned to behavioral items. We have included ICF codes for items that were not included.

### 3.2 Results of questionnaire evaluation of the Picotto system

The results of the questionnaire of the system to the research collaborators who used the system in 2016–2018 are shown in **Figure 5**. The total number of respondents to the questionnaire was 25: 10 parents, 7 teachers, 5 supporters, and 3 others.

About 70% of the users responded that they were able to share information with teachers, parents, and supporters and were able to see the child's behavior in concrete terms. In general, the use of the system was found to be effective. About 70% of the users thought that the introduction function of the support device service was effective. The chart function was used by only about 20% of the users. In the interview survey, there were requests to use the chart function for reports such as individual education support plans and reports, although it is not used much as a daily information sharing function.

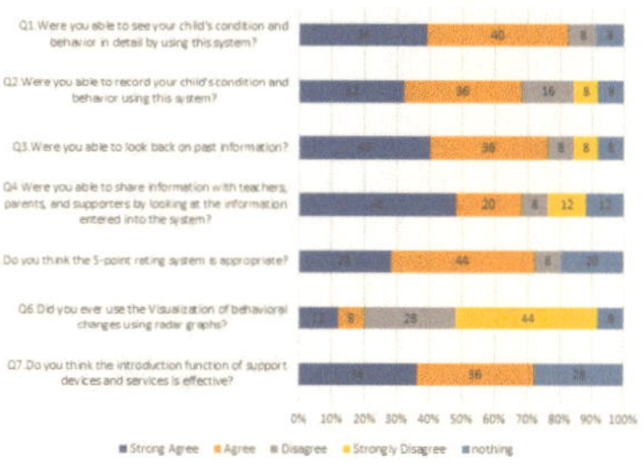


**Figure 5.**
*Results of questionnaire evaluation of the Picotto system.*

## 4. Introduction of support tools

Supportive services would be more effective if daily behavioral data were accumulated and analyzed in case conferences by homeroom teachers, parents, supporters, and specialists. Moreover, interventions using existing assistive devices will be used when available. However, if no suitable assistive devices are available, they can be developed. In our experience, it is better to conduct a needs survey for each person and individually develop equipment for that person, which often results in more user-friendly support-tools, rather than collecting the needs of many people and developing equipment because each person's developmental disabilities are different. We have found that it is better to develop several support-tools that meet individual needs, one by one, which will result in a product that meets everyone's needs, which is better than analyzing general needs and developing average support tools. Assistive devices have been developed based on individual characteristics and needs. For example, there are various assistive devices such as social skills training systems [13], support systems [14, 15], learning systems [16, 17], psychological tasks to examine personal characteristics [18, 19], etc. This chapter introduces several assistive technologies.

### 4.1 IoT support system using RFID, GPS

IoT technology is useful for locating people and things, such as "where are people?

Location-based services" are available to solve these problems. Speaking of location-based services, systems that utilize GPS (Global Positioning System) are already in use for managing people and objects moving over wide areas, and systems that use RFID (radio frequency identifier) are already in use for managing objects. In addition, GPS and RFID technologies have become very inexpensive to use. Therefore, they are being applied to the development of support tools to meet individual needs.

In this section, we explain the development process and usage of "Helping system not to forget anything using RFID" and "GPS Tracking System."

#### *4.1.1 Systems to help prevent lost and found items using RFID*

ADHD children often forget things. Forgetting things at school and other activities at school is a failure experience in daily life and often causes students to lose motivation. To continue to improve this, simply asking parents to check their children every day is not efficient, as well as losing the opportunity to check by themselves. Therefore, we developed a system to check for forgotten items by ourselves.

Register the timetable of each student and the information on belongings in the database of the system. If anomalous belongings, etc., increase due to change of schedule, etc., the teacher in charge of each student can add to belongings from the dedicated page. To use this system, paste the RFID tags on lecture notes and etc., students see the timetable and touch the necessary items on the tablet to check for forget items. Then, it checks with the database to check whether the ID assigned to RFID should be read and prepared. If there is a match, the color of the items that are displayed on the tablet is changed, visually as well, you can be sure that you are ready (**Figure 6**).

Children with developmental disorders also suffer from excessive anxiety over tasks that deviate from routine work. Therefore, the tablet terminal is fixed to the

*DOI: http://dx.doi.org/10.5772/intechopen.106065*

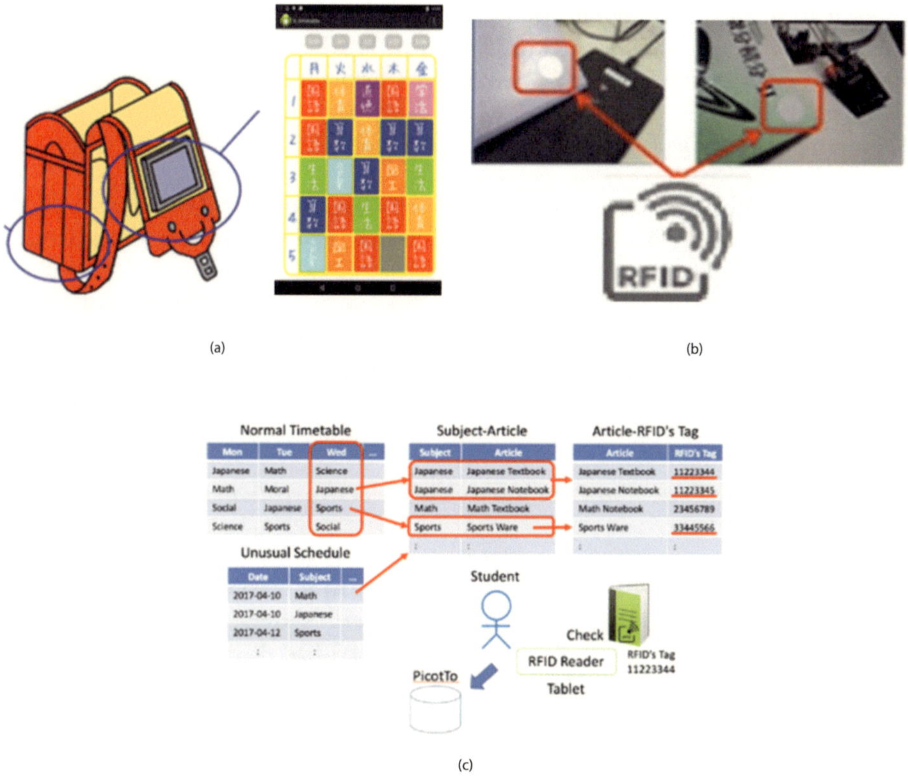


**Figure 6.**
*(a) Interface screen: tablet set in a school bag (b) RFID tags on textbook and notebook (c) database table structure.*

school bag, providing a tablet terminal, has been considered so that you do not have to take action, such as to prepare.

As a result, it is possible to focus only on the act of "match the timetable," there is no need to direct the useless attention.

User interface screens are developed according to the needs of the users, as they differ according to their requirements. For users who want to reduce the amount of information, we developed an interface screen that displays only one day's worth of information, and for users who want to grasp the entire schedule, we developed a weekly schedule.

### *4.1.2 GPS tracking system to school and home*

The prototype system was developed to manage school arrival and departure due to the need to know where they are when walking between school and home.

In order to take advantage of this feature, it is necessary to register the location information in advance. Here, the position information represents the latitude and longitude when dividing the road used at the time of going down and back school at intervals of several hundred meters. If students go through them in order, they can be regarded as going through prescribed roads. In order to start this tracking process, when students go to and from school, students do not need to operate tablets. You register your home and school in advance, and as soon as you leave a circle that is a few hundred meters in radius, tracking will start. Tracking will not start when you are staying in the circle of the specified two points (departure point and arrival point).

#### *4.1.3 Information sharing from assistive devices using API*

By sending information on students from IoT-based support devices, etc., to Picotto using API, information can be shared in real time with supporters at school, home, and professional organizations.

For example, if a student is able to go to school without deviating from the route, the five-point rating for the school attendance behavior item will be 5. Also, for example, if a student prepares three points of belongings, the behavior check item of the system will be given a three-point rating (**Figure** 7) (**Video 2**: https://youtu.be/14-chu1gh_M).

#### *4.1.4 Results of the IoT-based assistive devices questionnaire evaluation*

The results of a questionnaire survey of the system to research collaborators who used the system in 2016–2018 are shown in the **Figure 8**. Twenty-five people responded to the questionnaire: 10 parents, 7 teachers, 5 supporters, and 3 others

About half of the system users considered the GPS-based tracking system to be effective for school and home. More than 80% of the users wanted to use the system. About 70% of the respondents thought that the system to help prevent lost and found items using RFID was effective and wanted to use it. In addition, 60% of the users thought that the automatic collection of five-point evaluation values by the external linkage function was effective.

### 4.2 Plant pot system for communication support and living support

Plant cultivation has been reported to have a variety of positive effects on people, including relaxation and refreshment from the colors and fragrances, a sense of accomplishment from growth of plants, and daily exercise. In agriculture, the IoT is widely used and applied to cultivation management. We thought that the IoT

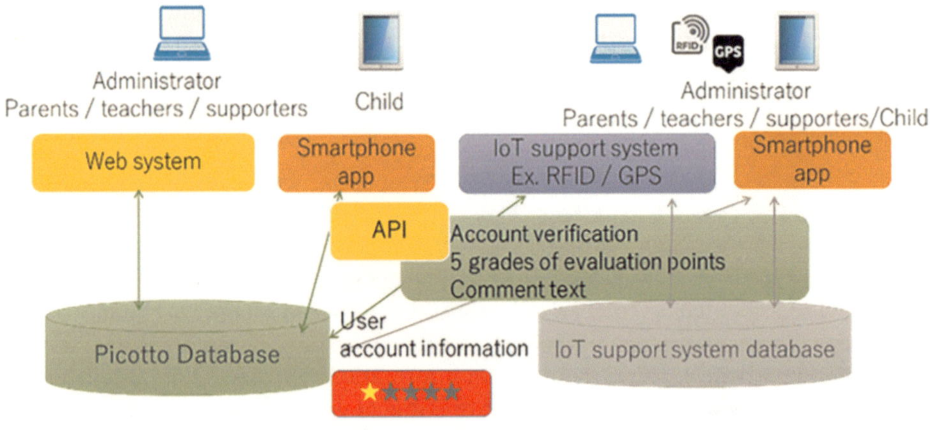


**Figure 7.**
*Collecting daily behavioral data of children with developmental disabilities from assistive devices and support services.*

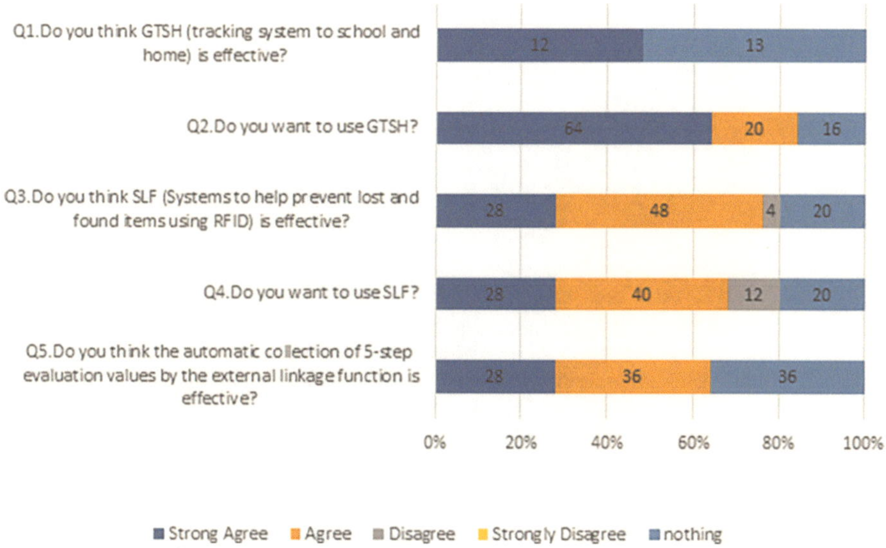


**Figure 8.**
*Results of the IoT-based assistive devices questionnaire evaluation.*

technology used in plant cultivation could be used not only for plant cultivation but also for supporting human life and communication and devised a plant pot that supports the daily life of the person cultivating the plants [20].

By using this system, we expect the following effects (1) and (2).

1. The system supports plant cultivation by collecting information on the surrounding environment using various sensors installed in the flowerpots and telling the user to adjust the temperature, solar radiation, and water content to suit the plant. The goal is to support the user's employment by providing a sense of accomplishment through plant cultivation while communicating with the system.

2. The system understands the user's daily rhythm based on the temperature and illumination information acquired by various sensors and the time of day and provides daily life support. The plant pot system recommends the use of air conditioning and heating to achieve the appropriate temperature for a person with sensory deprivation or encourages sleeping and waking for a person whose bedtime rhythm is disrupted.

The plant pot system contains wish of improvement and enhancement of our lives to be filled with smiles, that's why we named this pot "Etubo-chan," which means smiling pot in Japanese. **Figure 9** shows a photograph of this system. M5Stack Basic, which has a small display, speaker, SD card slot, and Wi-Fi communication, was used as the core microcomputer of the system. M5Stack Basic has a micro-SD card and stores Japanese character data and images of anthropomorphic plant pot characters. The character normally displays a sleeping image, and when the user approaches the plant pot system, the infrared sensor reacts and displays an image of the awakened character. At the same time, M5Stack outputs audio and text greetings that match the time obtained from the NTP server. If the time is past the preset bedtime, the system

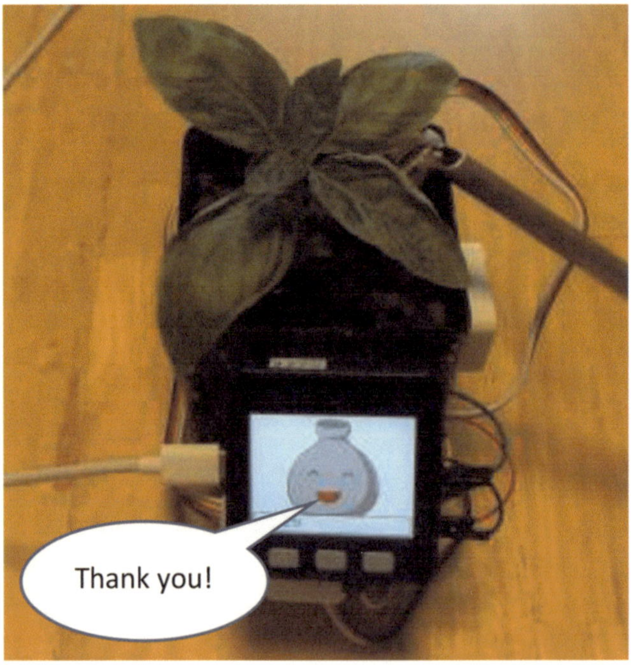


**Figure 9.**
*The plant pot system "Etubo-chan" (**Video 3**: https://youtu.be/TR7sVo1Kfug).*

outputs "I'm sleepy" to encourage the user to go to bed. Then, the system converses with the user to create an appropriate environment for the plant and human by using the values obtained from the illuminance sensor and the temperature/humidity/barometric pressure sensor. Specifically, the system outputs "It's too dark" when the illumination level is low and "It's too hot/cold" when the temperature is too hot/cold to encourage the user to take action. If the plants need water based on the soil moisture sensor value, the system tells them "I want water" and encourages watering. Finally, the system says on behalf of plants "thank you for coming see and watering me." In addition, the values of various sensors every 5 minutes, the time when a person approaches, and the time when watering is performed are saved in CSV format on a MicroSD card. **Video 1** (https://youtu.be/h8ekbDrvqhY) shows an example of the plant pot system working.

We conducted a verification experiment regarding the relaxation effect of this system. In the experiment, 12 subjects were asked to perform three tasks: Task A "watering a empty plant pot," Task B "watering a plant pot with a plant," and Task C "watering a plant pot system with a plant." At that time, EEG measurements and interviews were conducted. The alpha wave occupancy of each task was calculated from the EEG, and the averages of all of them were compared in **Figure 10**. The results showed that the occupancy of alpha waves during Task C "watering a plant pot system with a plant" was significantly higher than that during rest and Task A "watering a empty plant pot." This result suggests that the flowerpot system has a relaxing effect. In addition, in the interview survey, the participants commented that the flowerpot system "made them happy to talk," "the presence of the character made watering feel more meaningful," and "the system was cute and relaxed." In this study, we have developed a flowerpot system with a relaxing effect, and we received many positive comments.

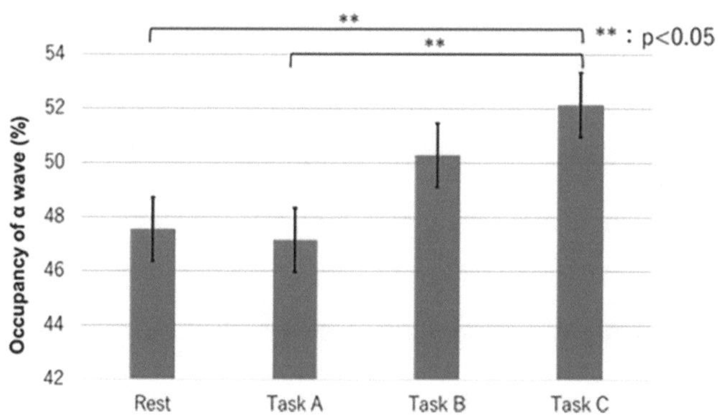


**Figure 10.**
*Comparison of the average α wave occupancy in each task.*

### 4.3 Programming education system and mentor training program for children with developmental disabilities

In Japan, there is a shortage of IT human resources, and as a national policy, programming education has been made mandatory in elementary, junior high, and high schools, with the aim of promoting the spread of programming education among young people.

However, the shortage of instructors to provide programming education is also a serious problem. Therefore, it is important to train IT personnel and instructors at universities and other institutions of higher education.

On the other hand, employment support for people with developmental disabilities is a pressing issue for the nation, and there are high expectations for IT workers because they can work from home even if they have disabilities, allowing them to work in a variety of ways.

Some developmentally disabled people with ASD are good at systemization [21], and we worked on programming education and training of educators (mentor training) for young developmentally disabled people aged 7–18 as a project commissioned by Japan's Ministry of Internal Affairs and Communications.

#### *4.3.1 Training mentors*

The characteristics of people with developmental disabilities vary from person to person in a hundred different ways, and it is important to understand developmental disabilities as well as to provide correct support. Furthermore, it is necessary for supporters of developmental disabilities to understand programming education and programming work.

Therefore, we planned a training program consisting of 15 lecturers (five people consisting of specialists in developmental disabilities, doctors, and educators, five IT professionals, five specialists who support employment for people with developmental disabilities), each lasting 30–60 minutes, with the aim of training mentors. The training sessions were videotaped, and e-Learning materials were created, making it possible to conduct mentor training on an ongoing basis regardless of location.

The mentors were teachers at special-needs schools and special-needs classes, undergraduate and graduate students in engineering, graduate students at technical colleges, undergraduate and graduate students in education, professional staff at after-school daycare services, and professional staff at temporary daytime support providers.

### *4.3.2 Mentor training course to understand development disabilities*

Mentor training course is largely divided into (1–3) fields with 30–60min lectures per segment.

1. **Course list relating to understanding people with developmental disabilities**

    - Psychological characteristics of developmental disabilities and educational support
    - Treatment of and rehabilitation for autism spectrum disorder, ADHD, and learning disabilities
    - Support for ASD in and out of school
    - Understand secondary disability in development disability
    - Focus on support for children with developmental disabilities at school and involvement with others

2. **Course list relating to science/manufacturing, programming education**

    - School course guidelines
    - Programming teaching materials
    - Programming educational methods corresponding to individual characteristics of children with developmental disabilities
    - Job as programmer
    - Integrated system development

3. **Employment support for people with developmental disabilities**

    - Support people with developmental disabilities with self-understanding
    - Employment of severely disabled people at home and coordination with special-needs school
    - A gap between education and labor
    - Anecdotal report of support for children with developmental disabilities
    - Inclusive society and science technology to realize it

#### *4.3.3 Development of new programming teaching materials based on characteristics of disabilities and implementation of programming education*

Computer programming is considered an important skill for developing higher-order thinking in addition to algorithmic problem-solving skills, and there are high expectations for the development of mathematical concepts and problem-solving skills [22], such as Scratch [23] and Scratch Jr [24], which is specialized for young learners. With the advent of computer programming tools with visual design for beginners, programming education using such tools has been popular in Japan.

Our target learners this time are students at special-needs schools and students with developmental disabilities receiving after-school day care services or temporary daytime support. In the past, we have held classes using general-purpose programming development tools such as Scratch, but because tools such as Scratch are multifunctional, they are difficult for these children with disabilities, and they often lose track of what to do. Therefore, we developed programming materials to foster logical thinking, such as various commands (walk, change direction, conditional branching, and repetition) through visual design, with the goal of solving clear-cut tasks such as escaping from a maze. The program is cloud-based and can be learned anytime, anywhere.

The programming materials were devised to enable children with developmental disabilities to work on them with interest and perseverance, taking into account their characteristics as follows.

Programming teaching materials were designed based on the following rule of SPELL. Further, curricula and methods of instruction were examined based on the rule.

1. **Designing programming teaching materials based on the rule of SPELL**

    - Structure: Set up easy and clear framework

        - Develop visualized and structured teaching materials

    - Positive: Get involved positively (praise)

        - Give praise for success

    - Emphasis: Empathy (understand)

        - Give encouragement even if failed

    - Low arousal: Low stimulation as excessive stimulation would cause panic by preparing eye-friendly screen layout conducive to working with calm, students who take the course can select screen layout of their liking (**Figure 11**).

    - Links: Bond (connection with community, mentors and students, and peers, cooperation)

Provide an opportunity to facilitate communication by using projection mapping for testing program operations

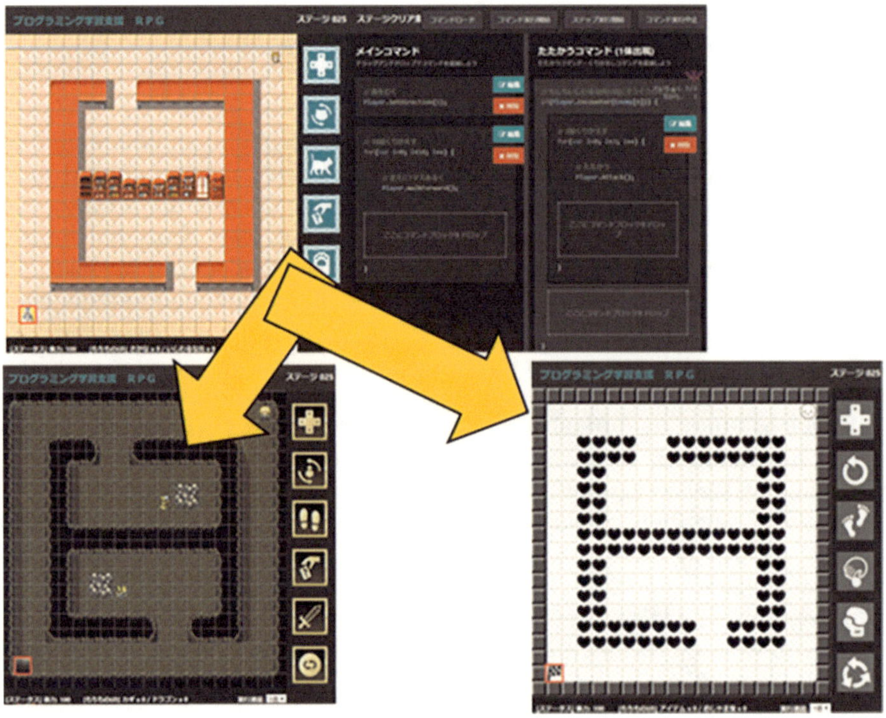

**Figure 11.**
*Children can choose the favorite screen layout according to their personal characteristics.*

### 2. Ingenuity in programming teaching materials based on characteristics of disabilities

User interface with assist features by taking the characteristics of people with developmental disabilities into consideration.

User interface with assist features by taking the characteristics of people with developmental disabilities into consideration

- "Give praise" when program operation goes well.

- "Mollify" and "give hints" when not operating.

Understand sequential executions and control structures (repetition, conditional branching) with visual design and feel the concept of event-driven, and so on (**Figure 12**).

**Figure 13** is a screen shot of one stage (Stage006). The pop-up window on the right of the figure shows a clear goal. The cat character near the center of the maze is trying to reach the goal at the bottom while avoiding obstacles. Hints are given such as combining the "direction," "repeat," and "walk" commands.

- When Start, Goal is completed with simulation operation, a praising mark appears.

- Even if fails, give encouragement with just a bit more mark.

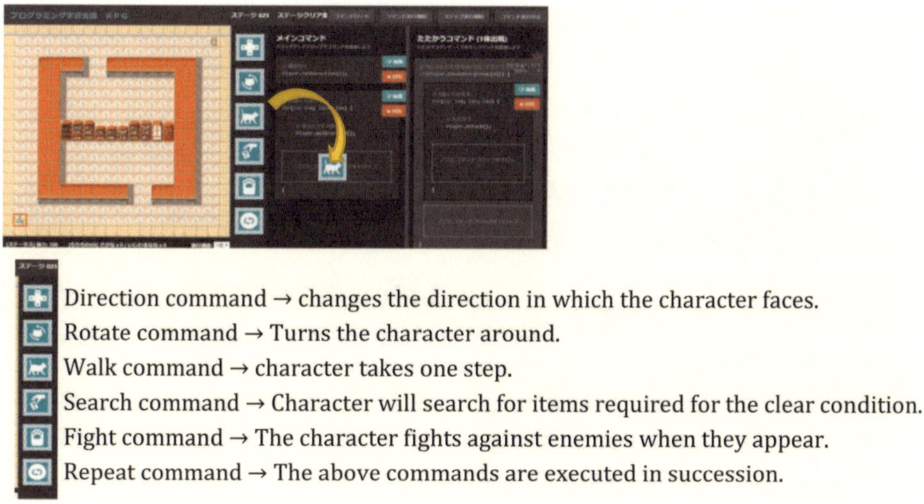


**Figure 12.**
*Programming creation tool with visual design (explanation of each command).*

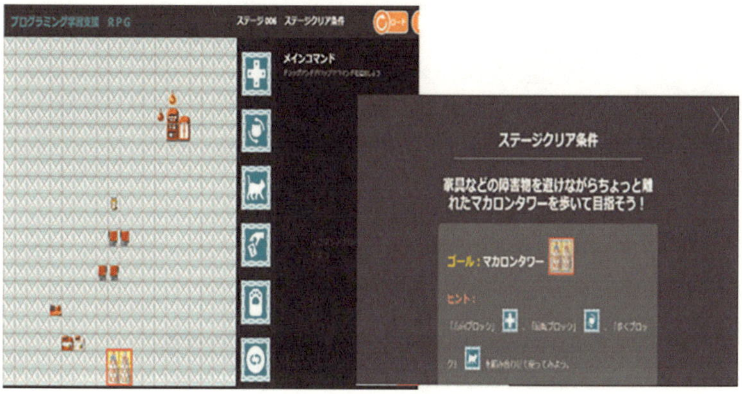


**Figure 13.**
*Maze assignment with clear goals.*

- Work on the challenge of escaping from a maze by a virtual robot with a clear goal.
- The aim is simple and clear.
- Ponder an effective path to reach a goal in maze escape game.

The aim is simple and clear. Ponder an effective path to reach a goal in maze escape game.

Programming becomes possible by combining commands with visual design and inputting parameter in the command (**Figure 14**). Each command block can be shifted to Java source for learning coding (**Figure 15**).

**Figure 16** shows the image when the command is executed. You can also check the operation while executing the command (source code) on the right side of the screen step by step.

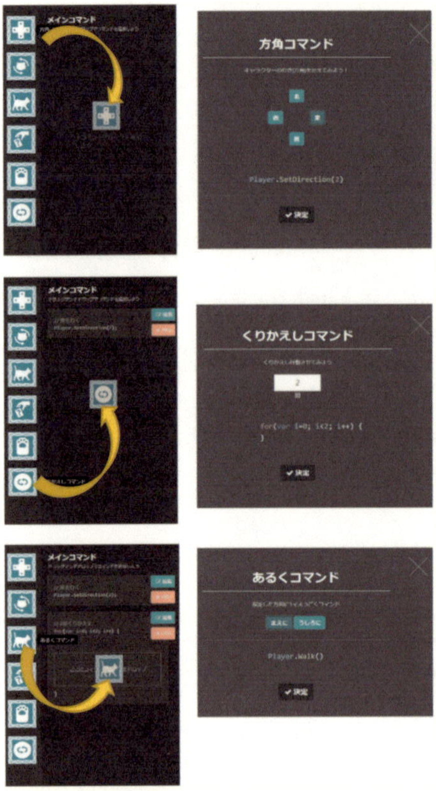


Drop direction command.
A pop-up window will then appear to select the direction.

Select "East" and press the "Decide" button.

Next, drop the repeat command.

A pop-up window for entering the number of repetitions will then appear.

Enter a value of "2" in the text box and press the "Decide" button.

Next, drop the walk command into the repeat command.

A pop-up window will then appear to determine the direction of the walk command.

Select the "Walk Forward" button and press the Decide button.

**Figure 14.**
*An example of programming work.*

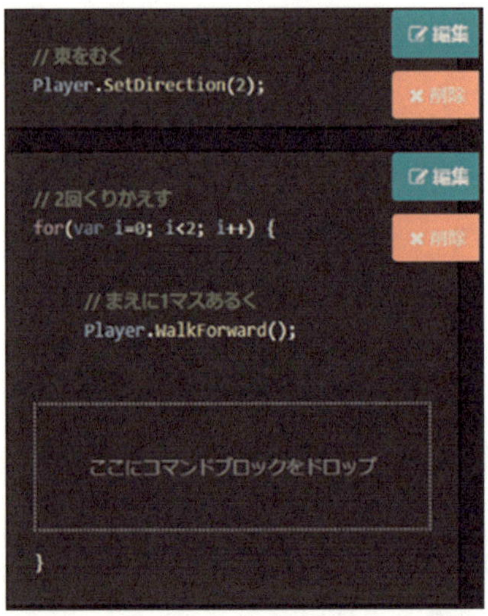


**Figure 15.**
*Java source code for command buttons.*

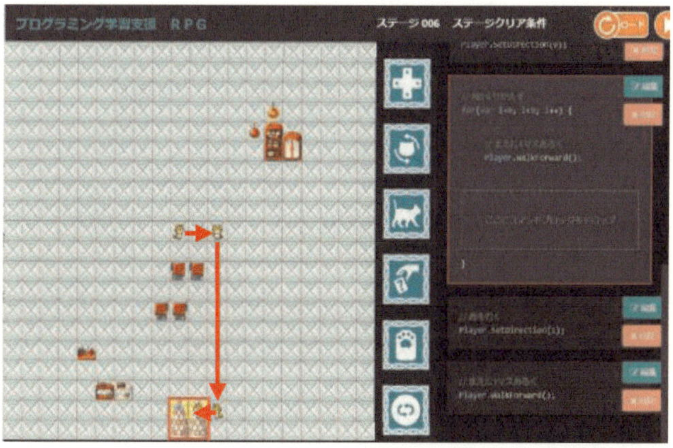

**Figure 16.**
*Execution of commands.*

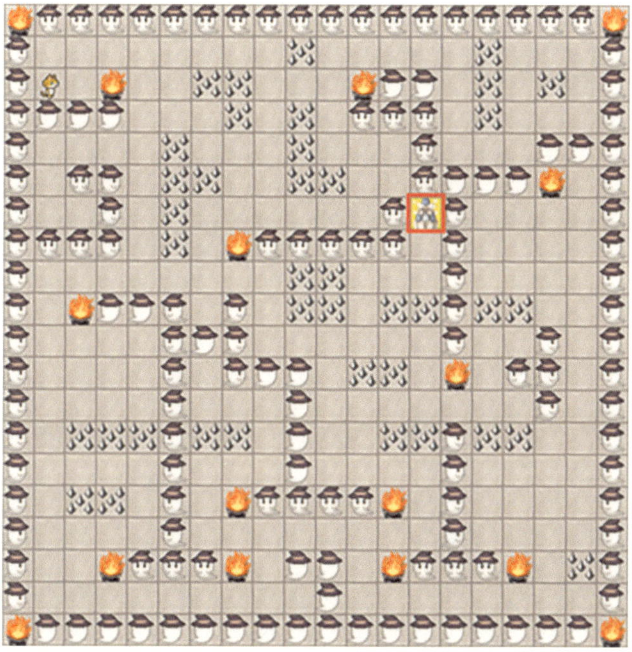

**Figure 17.**
*An example of a difficult stage (Stage 20).*

A total of 30 kinds of stages were set up with the difficulty level gradually going up. Formulate a plan such as getting treasures to earn points (**Figure 17**).

While operations can be checked individually in the computer terminal, offer a favorable environment for interacting each other using projection mapping via 3DG on a table with students around it (**Figure 18**).

As for projection mapping, the stereographic projection is used from both right and left, so as not to cast a shadow. Direct input is also planned by using pointing device.

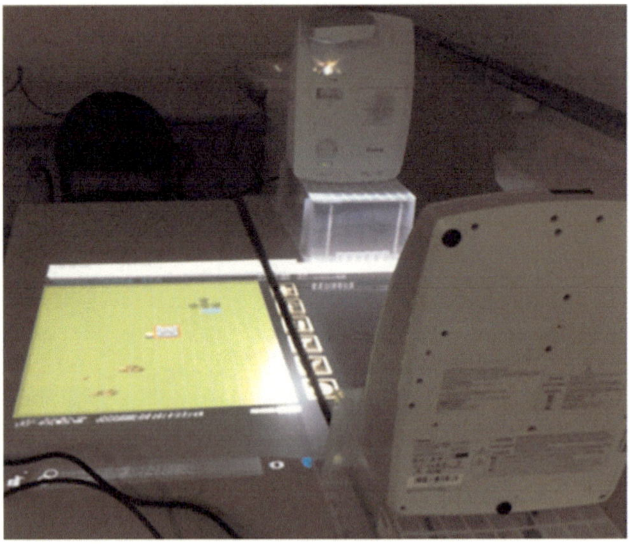

**Figure 18.**
*Execution screen of programming material using projection mapping.*

Take the status of disabilities and the characteristics of children and students into consideration and do a follow-up.

The progress of students working on the challenge of programming can be grasped in the server, which can be utilized by professionals and mentors in conducting individualized teaching.

#### *4.3.4 The status of programming class*

A programming class was conducted at five schools so far, involving 24 students who took the course and 20 mentors.

We conducted a model class the first time and mentors took the lead in continuing to conduct programming class the second time and thereafter. A view of the classroom is shown in **Figure 19**.

Especially, children with intellectual disabilities could understand aims and command details, went ahead with formulating programming, and managed to advance several stages.

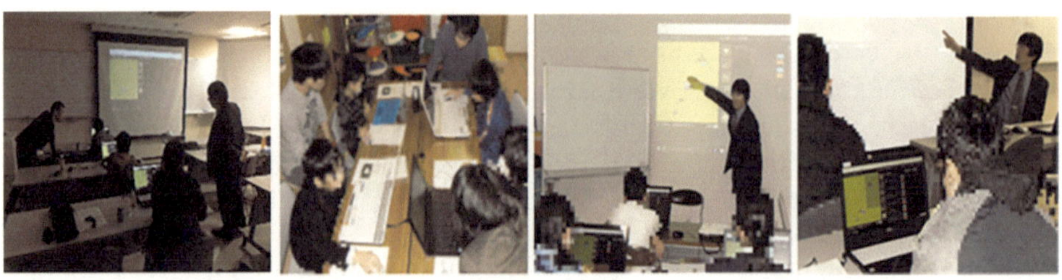

**Figure 19.**
*Programming class.*

A person specialized in supporting people with developmental disabilities but not in programming commented that "I could also use teaching materials like these for teaching."

While working on the task, even children with autistic tendencies showed behaviors such as teaching their peers. There is an evaluation report of peer tutoring as a means of aiding the learning of programming languages [25]. This is not only effective for learning, but also provides an opportunity to promote communication, and peer tutoring may play an important role, especially for ASD children who have difficulty with communication.

#### *4.3.5 Questionnaire results*

(1) Training mentors

The composition of the mentors who participated in the project was characterized by a high percentage of those with programming experience (**Figure 20**).

Approximately 90% (19 out of 21) of the mentors indicated that the programming courses were implemented as planned (**Figure 21**).

The areas that were successfully implemented and those that were not are shown in **Figures 22** and **23**, respectively.

(2) Results of questionnaire on programming courses

From the implementer's free answer:

- I think that the programming materials developed were able to clarify the issues and their objectives very well. The programming materials we developed were able to clarify the tasks and their objectives very well.

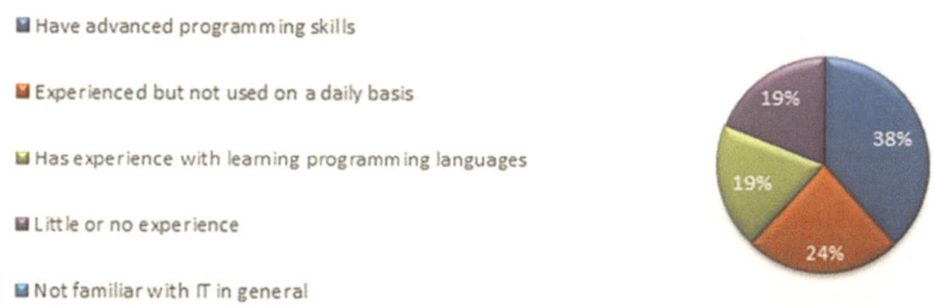


**Figure 20.**
*Mentor's background (programming skills).*

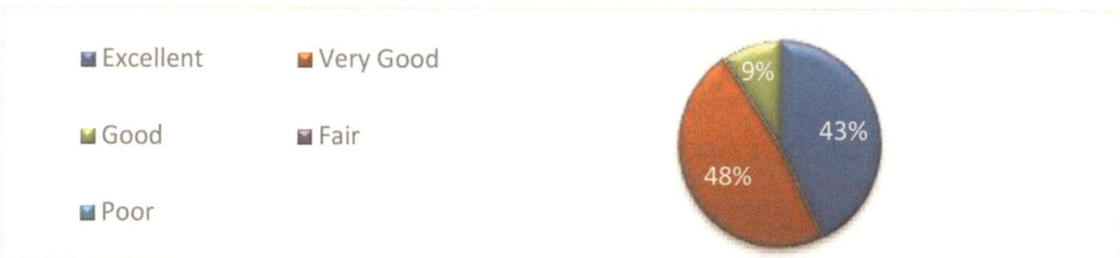


**Figure 21.**
*Whether the course was accomplished as planned.*

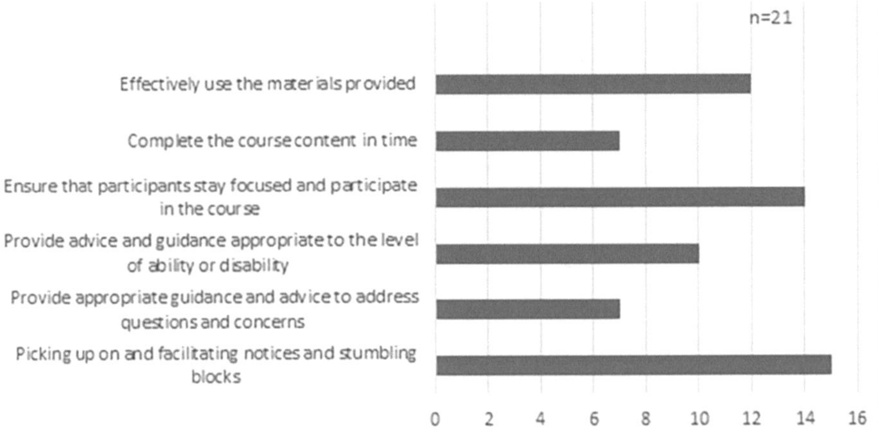


**Figure 22.**
*Questionnaire results on areas that were successfully implemented.*

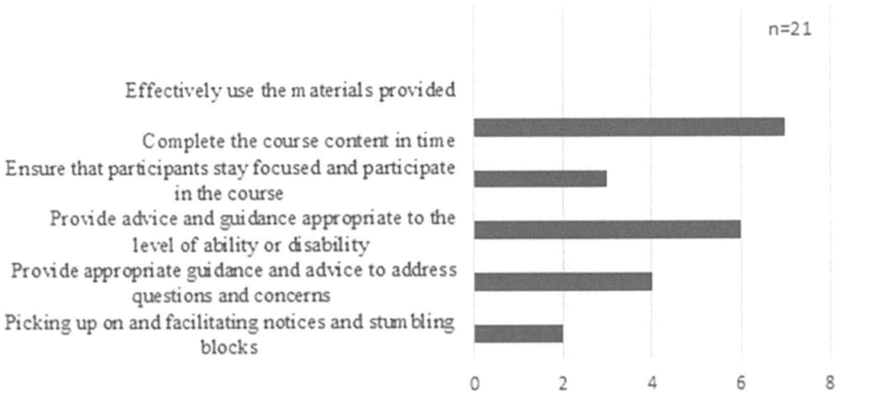


**Figure 23.**
*Questionnaire results regarding areas that were not implemented well.*

- The control structures such as sequential execution, repetition and conditional branching, which are indispensable elements of programming, were relatively easy to understand. This was a success beyond our expectations.

- The students were able to easily understand the operations of buttons, etc., which are necessary to build up programming (to give commands).

- In order to solve the given task, logical thinking, i.e., thinking about the order and combination of various commands, is necessary. This was a success beyond our expectations.

- The scope of instruction was clearly defined based on an understanding of the children's aptitudes.

- The preparation of the PC environment was very smooth.

- It was good that the children showed interest in programming.

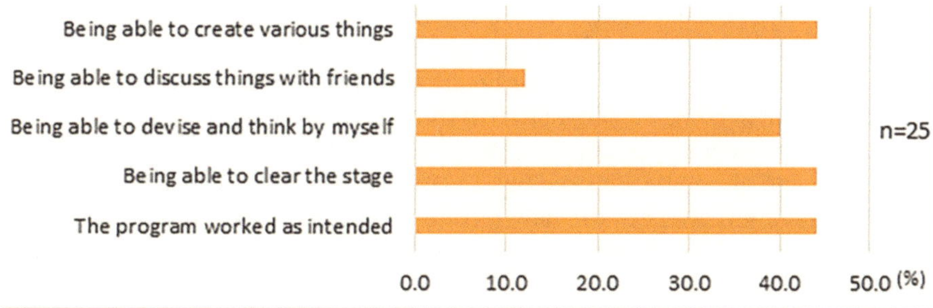


**Figure 24.**
*Results of a survey on the reasons why "programming" was interesting.*

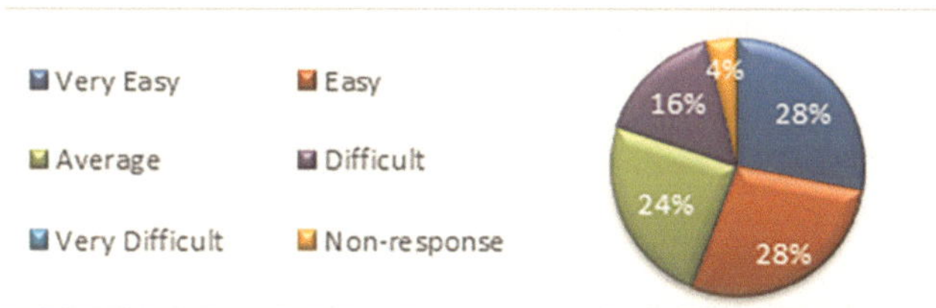


**Figure 25.**
*Whether the lecture content and exercises were difficult or not.*

From the pupils' questionnaires:

- The students found programming interesting in terms of character movement and completing stages, as well as in their own devising and experimenting (**Figure 24**).

Regarding the contents explained by the mentors and what they actually did, 14 out of 25 students answered that it was easy, while four students answered that it was a little difficult, indicating that the degree of difficulty varied from person to person.

The fact that 80% of the students (20 out of 25) answered that the contents and use of the course materials was easy to understand indicates that the course materials were easy to use for most of the students (**Figure 25**).

## 5. Summary and future issues

In this study, it was found that support for children with developmental disabilities using an ICT-based system for immediate information sharing among support schools, families, and specialized institutions was effective. In the results of the questionnaire, the system's functions were generally highly evaluated. Contrary to expectations, the visualization of behavioral changes using radar graphs function was not used very often. This may be because both teachers and parents can grasp the situation of their children by viewing daily behavioral data. However, there was a desire to use the radar graphs to create reports on individualized educational support plans. In the future, we would like to develop a function that makes it possible to compose reports on individualized educational support plans in an easier-to-understand manner.

In Japan today, various changes in social structure are taking place with the new Corona, Society 5.0, the GIGA school concept, DX, etc. In particular, the Corona disaster has promoted the use of IT in schools, and now that the infrastructure for one device per student is being established, this trend is expected to accelerate.

Therefore, the most important thing for this project is to analyze the results while implementing and giving back to society. In the fast-paced IT field, it is important to quickly introduce and adapt to the new technology while putting it into actual use, and it is necessary to keep a fast spiral and not overlook the sense of difficulty of a minority group.

Therefore, the goal is to construct a system that is adapted to society by paying attention to social trends and collaborating with researchers from various fields, especially humanities and social sciences researchers, engineering researchers, and teachers in the field. Human-centered design is conducted to identify the needs of students and families, the school management system, and the needs of the field. Then, we will clarify the mechanisms of educational support and welfare support and their issues and propose and construct a feasible and sustainable support system. Currently, the PoC is being conducted with the cooperation of the Fukui Prefecture Teachers' Union. The current issue is the busy schedules of teachers and parents, and we are developing a system that can centralize duplicated tasks to solve the busy schedules of teachers and parents while providing effective support for students. We hope that the educational system and the system will cooperate with each other, leading to a society in which no one is left behind, for all students and their parents.

We want to realize close, efficient, and collaborative support in time for students to enter society, so that they can live and work in society without suffering, and so that they can lead a better life and have more opportunities to learn. We believe that ICT individualized educational support system will play a role in making education more effective in today's busy society.

## Acknowledgements

This work was supported by JSPS KAKENHI Grant Number JP18K02896・JP19K12245・JP22K02786・JP22K12283, and SCOPE:162305008.

## Notes/thanks/other declarations

We would like to thank the Fukui Teachers' Union, teachers in Fukui Prefecture, parents, supporters, and collaborators.

**Author details**

Sakiko Ogoshi[1*], Yasuhiro Ogoshi[2], Tohru Saitoh[1], Kotoko Tanaka[3], Yoichi Itoh[4], Masahiro Wakamatu[4], Tomoyuki Kanno[4] and Akio Nakai[5]

1 National Institute of Technology, Fukui College, Sabae, Fukui, Japan

2 Graduate School of Engineering, University of Fukui, Fukui, Fukui, Japan

3 University of Fukui, Fukui, Fukui, Japan

4 Hitachi Solutions East Japan Ltd., Sendai, Miyagi, Japan

5 Graduate School of Clinical Education and The Center for the Study of Child Development, Institute for Education, Mukogawa Women's University, Hyogo, Japan

*Address all correspondence to: ogoshi@fukui-nct.ac.jp

## References

[1] Polanczyk G, de Lima MS, Horta BL, Biederman J, Rohde LA. The worldwide prevalence of ADHD: A systematic review and metaregression analysis. The American Journal of Psychiatry. 2007; **164**(6):942-948

[2] Hertz-Picciotto I, Delwiche L. The rise in autism and the role of age at diagnosis. Epidemiology. 2009;**20**(1): 84-90

[3] Nassar N, Dixon G, Bourke J, Bower C, Glasson E, de Klerk N, et al. Autism spectrum disorders in young children: Effect of changes in diagnostic practices. International Journal of Epidemiology. 2009;**38**(5):1245-1254

[4] Altarac M, Saroha E. Lifetime prevalence of learning disability among US children. Pediatrics. 2007;**119**:S77-S83

[5] Georgia D, Flouris AD, Yiannis K, Brent EF, Alan MN, Andrew ML, et al. A comparison of developmental coordination disorder prevalence rates in Canadian and Greek Children. Journal of Adolescent Health. 2006;**39**(1):125-127

[6] Lingam R, Hunt L, Golding J, Jongmans M, Emond A. Prevalence of developmental coordination disorder using the DSM-IV at 7 years of age: A UK Population Based Study. Pediatrics. 2009;**123**(4):e693-e700

[7] Recent Policy and Status on Special Needs Education in Japan. NISE Bulletin. 2019

[8] Crowe B, Machalicek W, Wei Q, Drew C, Ganz J. Augmentative and alternative communication for children with intellectual and developmental disability: A mega-review of the literature. Journal of Developmental and Physical Disabilities. 2022;**34**(1):1-42

[9] Somabut A, Tuamsuk K. Online Teaching and Learning Ecology in Thai Higher Education during the COVID-19 Pandemic. London, UK: Intechopen. p. 100222

[10] Mark Tomlinson M, Yasamy T, Emerson E, Officer A, Richler D, Saxena S. Setting global research priorities for developmental disabilities, including intellectual disabilities and autism. Journal of Intellectual Disabililities and Autism. 2014;**58**(12): 1121-1130

[11] Tokunaga Y. Support for Persons with Developmental Disabilities in Japan. Japan: NISE Bulletin, National Institute of Special Needs Education; 2014

[12] World Health Organization. International Classification of Functioning, Disability and Health (ICF). Available from: http://www.who.int/classifications/icf/en/

[13] Takezawa T, Ogoshi S, Ogoshi Y, Mitsuhashi Y, Hiratani M. Computer based training program to facilitate learning of the relationship between facial-based and situation-based emotions and prosocial behaviors. Industrial Engineering and Management Systems. 2012;**11**(2):142-147

[14] Ogoshi S, Ogoshi Y, Saitou T, Nishi H, Mituhasi Y, Nakai A. Development of sleep support system using electroencephalogram for person with developmental disabilities. Sensors and Materials. 2018;**30**(7): 1457-1462

[15] Ogoshi Y, Ogoshi S, Emoto A. Development of an education support system for children with developmental

disabilities - Suggestion the special supported room using information technology. In: IEEE 10th International Conference on Engineering Education (ICEED). 2018. DOI: 10.1109/iceed.2018.8626897

[16] Ogoshi Y, Ogoshi S, Yamazaki K, Takezawa T, Nakai A, Tsuji K, et al. Expiration training system for treatment of people with speech problems. Sensors and Materials. 2014; **26**(7):519-528

[17] Ogoshi Y, Ogoshi S, Takezawa T, Mitsuhashi Y. Impact of the facial attractiveness of a social reward on event-related potential activities and task performance. Sensors and Materials. 2016;**28**(4):321-327

[18] Ogoshi S, Ogoshi Y, Momose S, Takezawa T, Mitsuhashi Y. Mu rhythm suppression during the imagination of observed action. In: Proceedings of the Annual International Conference of the IEEE Engineering in Medicine and Biology Society (EMBS). 2013. pp. 4310-4313

[19] Ogoshi S, Takezawa T, Ogoshi Y, Yanaka T, Mitsuhashi Y. Overview of social cognitive ability from the perspective of facial expressions and context-estimating emotion based on context essays and facial expressions. Sensors and Materials. 2014;**26**(7): 505-518

[20] Tanaka K, Ogoshi S, Shimada M, Ogoshi Y. Development of human friendly plant cultivation pot using IoT. In: IEEE International Conference on Consumer Electronics Taiwan (ICCE-TW). 2021. pp. 15-17

[21] Baron-Cohen S. The Essential Difference: Male and Female Brains and the Truth about Autism. New York: Basic Books; 2004

[22] Fessakis G, Gouli E, Mavroudi E. Problem solving by 5–6 years old kindergarten children in a computer programming environment: A case study. Computers & Education. 2013;**63**: 87-97

[23] Scratch. Available from: https://scratch.mit.edu

[24] Louise P, Silverman B, Kazakoff ER, Bers MU, Bontá P, Resnick M. Designing Scratch: Support for early childhood learning through computer programming. In: Proceedings of the 12th International Conference on Interaction Design and Children. 2013. pp. 1-10

[25] de la Hera DP, Zanoni MB, Sigman M, Calero CI. Peer tutoring of computer programming increases exploratory behavior in children. Journal of Experimental Child Psychology. 2022; **216**:1-18. DOI: 10.1016/j.jecp.2021.105335

Chapter 4

# Gestational Tryptophan Fluctuation Underlying Ontogenetic Origin of Neuropsychiatric Disorders

*Xiaohong Huang, Xiaohua Li and Heng-Wei Cheng*

## Abstract

Neuropsychiatry underlies personality development and social functioning. Borderline personality disorder exhibits high trait aggression and is associated with tryptophan hydroxylase polymorphisms. The acute tryptophan depletion reduces plasma and cerebrospinal fluid tryptophan availability and brain serotonin concentrations, leading to alterations in personality and trait-related behaviors. Tryptophan is essential for fatal neurodevelopment and immunomodulation in pregnancy. Gestational tryptophan fluctuation induced by maternal metabolic disorders or drug administrations may account for the maternal-fetal transmission determining neurogenesis and microbial development, consequentially shaping the long-standing patterns of thinking and behavior. However, it is not possible to assess the gestational tryptophan exposure effects on fetal brain and gastrointestinal system in humans for ethical reasons. The maternal–fetal microbe transmission in rodents during gestation, vaginal delivery, and breastfeeding is inevitable. Chicken embryo may be an alternative and evidence from the chicken embryo model reveals that gestational tryptophan fluctuation, i.e., exposed to excessive tryptophan or its metabolite, serotonin, attenuates aggressiveness and affects peer sociometric status. This chapter discusses the gestational tryptophan fluctuation as a risk factor of personality disorders in offspring and the prevention of personality disorders by dietary tryptophan control and medication therapy management during pregnancy.

**Keywords:** gestation, tryptophan, neuropsychiatry, neuroendocrine, microbiota-gut-brain axis

## 1. Introduction

Personality is mediated by multi-factors, including brain chemistry and life experiences, reflecting people's long-standing patterns of thinking and behavior [1]. Strong association between childhood adversity and a diagnosis of personality disorder in young adulthood has been revealed by a cohort study in 2017 among individuals born in Stockholm County [2]. Indeed, personality already starts in the womb, and prenatal experience influences temperament development [3]. A longitudinal birth cohort study in 2019 revealed the potential association between prenatal stress exposure and personality disorders in Finland [4]. However, scientifically plausible inferences regarding the causality are not assessable in view of those retrospective data. In the context that the evidence from prospective longitudinal studies supports early-life experience programming personality development, it is crucial to investigate how early-life stimuli cause personality disorders and relevant neurobiological mechanisms.

Borderline personality disorder (BPD, ICD-10-CM code F60.3) patients present high trait aggression [5], and BPD is associated with the polymorphism of tryptophan hydroxylase (TPH) 1 and TPH2 [6–8]. Tryptophan (Trp) is essential for fetal growth including neurodevelopment and immunomodulation in pregnancy [9]. Gestational Trp fluctuation caused by maternal metabolic disorders or drug administrations may account for the maternal-fetal transmission determining neurogenesis and microbial development, consequentially shaping the long-standing patterns of thinking and behavior in offspring [10–12]. Several current studies indicate that gestational Trp exposure yields bullying victim while exposed to excessive serotonin (5-hydroxytryptophan, 5-HT) reduces aggressiveness in bullies [11, 12]. Such studies improve our understanding of temperament development and hold the promise to promote advances in the preventing and treating personality disorders.

## 2. Ontogenetic origin of neuropsychiatric disorders

### 2.1 Neuropsychiatric basis of personality disorders

Personality has been broadly considered in neuropsychiatry and vice versa [13]. People with personality disorders have more rigid thinking and hyperreactive behaviors, which makes it hard for them to perceive and adapt to the surrounding situations and people. Patients with BPD display increased stress vulnerability, which is linked to the dysfunction of the hypothalamic-pituitary-adrenal (HPA) axis [14], with lower baseline cortisol levels compared with healthy controls [15]. The cortisol awakening response, presumed to mirror maladaptive neuroendocrine processes, is increased in female individuals with BPD [14]. Moreover, the role of cortisol and testosterone in regulating aggressive and socially dominant behavior in children and adults has been proposed by the dual-hormone hypothesis [16], suggesting the involvement of the hypothalamic-pituitary-gonadal (HPG) axis also. The first evidence from mixed-sex community adolescents reveals that the joint effects of testosterone and cortisol on externalizing problems, which is especially pronounced in individuals with disagreeableness and emotional instability personality pathology traits [16]. Hence, the development and activity of the neuroendocrine system lay the foundation of personality traits. And, the link between personality traits and neurodevelopmental disorders (NDDs) has been explored by Child and Adolescent Twin Study in Sweden (CATSS), such as attention deficit hyperactivity disorder (ADHD, ICD-10 codes F90) and autism spectrum disorder (ASD, ICD-10 code F84.0) [13]. The character dimensions of cooperativeness and self-directedness and ASD are negatively correlated and ADHD alike [13].

### 2.2 Maternal-fetal transmission in ontogenetic origin of neuropsychiatric disorders

Barker's hypothesis proposes the ontogenetic origin of adult diseases [17]. Maternal malnutrition or drug administration altering maternal metabolism influences fetal development through maternal-fetal transmission. The correlation between maternal 5-HT levels and offspring cognitive ability has been identified in ASD [18]. A nationwide cohort study in France found that increased NDDs occurrence is associated with gestational exposure to valproate, an antiepileptic drug [19]. Moreover, antenatal valproate exposure induces changes and abnormalities in the gastrointestinal microstructure and function in rats, indicated by the thinned tunica mucosa and tunica muscularis of the ileum [20]. The changes parallel the gastrointestinal symptoms in ASD patients [20]. Moreover, patients with ASD have significant changes in the gut microbiome, e.g., increased abundance of family *Sutterellaceae* and *Enterobacteriaceae* and decreased abundance of genus *Bifidobacterium* [21]. Hence, maternal metabolic fluctuation may directly interfere fetal neurogenesis and/or indirectly reprogram gut microbial development to alter the function of the microbiota-gut-brain (MGB) axis with the potential for neuropsychiatric disorders in offspring.

## 3. Tryptophan in pregnancy

Tryptophan, an essential amino acid, is critical for pregnancy attributing to fetal neurogenesis and immunomodulation [9]. Tryptophan is the sole precursor of 5-HT [22]. Maternal circuiting Trp takes part in fetal brain development via the 5-HT pathway regulating synaptogenesis and neuronal maturation, e.g., the thalamocortical pathfinding is disrupted by modifying the 5-HT abundance in the embryonic mouse brain [23]. Tryptophan is synthesized into 5-HT in the placenta and delivered to the fetal brain or delivered directly to the fetal brain, then synthesized into 5-HT [22]. Two BPD risk factors, i.e., the 5-HT 1A receptor promoter polymorphism (rs6295) and dopamine (DA) transporter repeat allele, have been identified in 367 patients with major depressive disorders (MDDs) [24]. Another metabolic pathway of placental Trp is degradation along the cytokine-induced activated Trp catabolite (TRYCAT) pathway, producing kynurenines (KYNs) to suppress T cell responses [25]. A disturbed TRYCAT pathway in the fetal brain has been characterized in people with schizophrenia (ICD-10 code F20.9), a neurodevelopmental disorder [26]. Low plasma concentrations of Trp and KYN have been found in patients with severe anxiety and depression during pregnancy [27] while excess Trp causes preeclampsia (ICD-10-CM code O14.90), which results in long-term endocrine morbidity in offspring [28]. Preeclampsia has been associated with increased NDDs occurrence, including ASD, ADHD, mental retardation (ICD-10 code F70–F79), epilepsy (ICD-10 code G40) [29]. Both the increases in maternal urinary Trp concentration and ASD risk of offspring have been seen in gestational diabetes mellitus (ICD-10-CM code O24.419) patients [30, 31]. Moreover, antenatal stress adversely affects neurodevelopment via disrupting placental Trp metabolism, laying the neurobiological foundation of psychiatric disorders [32]. The gut Trp-metabolizing microbes, i.e., the genera *Parasutterella* and *Bifidobacterium*, are reduced in the dam and offspring following prenatal maternal stress [33]. Thus, malnutrition and drug administrations during pregnancy may have altered placental Trp availability, the function of TRYCAT pathway, and/or the abundance of gut Trp-metabolizing microbes, leading to neuropsychiatric disorders in offspring.

## 4. Tryptophan and personality traits

### 4.1 Tryptophan hydroxylase polymorphisms in personality traits and disorders

Tryptophan hydroxylases (TPHs), the rate-limiting enzymes, convert Trp into 5-HT at the different locations, i.e., TPH1 in the body and TPH2 in the brain [22]. The polymorphisms within TPH genes, involved in regulating the Trp–5-HT conversion, are relevant to personality traits and disorders. The relationship between TPH single-nucleotide polymorphisms (SNPs) and personality traits/disorders has been reviewed in **Table 1**. For example, rs1800532 is associated with trait emotional intelligence [34], anger-related traits [35, 36], antisocial personality disorder [39], and BPD [6]. However, negative results have been reported in other studies [37, 38]. The controversy may be caused by the sampling population or sample size. And, it may be resolved by the involvement of other SNPs, i.e., haplotype [7, 8]. For example, a TPH2 "risk" haplotype (rs2171363, rs6582078, rs1352250) has been identified in a well-characterized clinical sample of 251 patients with personality disorders and 103 healthy controls, associated with BPD diagnosis, affective lability, and aggression [8].

| Gene | Sample | Single nucleotide polymorphism | Personality trait/ disorder | Ref. |
|---|---|---|---|---|
| TPH1 | 336 healthy Korean college students | rs1800532 | Trait emotional intelligence | [34] |
| | 251 community-derived volunteers in Pittsburgh | rs1800532 | Anger-related traits and aggression | [35] |
| | 544 suicide attempters in Switzerland | rs1800532 | Anger-related traits | [36] |
| | 345 Japanese healthy subjects | rs1800532 | Not associated with personality traits | [37] |
| | 228 healthy Korean women | rs1800532 | Not associated with anger-related traits | [38] |
| | 310 participants with antisocial personality disorder and 200 with no antisocial personality disorder | rs1800532 | Antisocial personality disorder | [39] |
| | 100 patients diagnosed with borderline personality disorder and 101 non-psychiatric controls | rs1800532 | Borderline personality disorder | [6] |
| | 86 suicide attempters and 154 community-based healthy volunteers in German | rs1800532, rs1799913 | Anger-related traits | [40] |
| | Caucasian students of German ancestry without any history of psychopathology or drug abuse: 108 smokers and 144 nonsmokers | rs1799913 | Neurotic aggression | [41] |
| | 253 healthy Japanese subjects | rs1799913 | Not associated with personality traits | [42] |
| | 95 Caucasian women with borderline personality disorder had attempted suicide at least twice during their lifetime and 98 women without psychiatric history | rs4537731, rs684302, rs211105, rs1800532, rs1799913, rs7933505 | Borderline personality disorder | [7] |

| Gene | Sample | Single nucleotide polymorphism | Personality trait/ disorder | Ref. |
|---|---|---|---|---|
| TPH2 | 1176 Estonian subjects | rs4570625 | Adaptive impulsivity and trait anxiety | [43] |
| | 228 healthy Korean women | rs4570625 | Anger-related traits | [38] |
| | 1576 Estonian teenagers | rs4570625 | Neuroticism and conscientiousness | [44] |
| | 63 healthy Korean women | rs4570625 | Anger-related traits | [45] |
| | 336 healthy volunteers of German descent | rs4570625 | Anxiety-related traits | [46] |
| | 251 patients with personality disorders and 103 healthy controls | rs2171363, rs6582078, rs1352250 | Borderline personality disorder and aggression | [8] |

**Table 1.**
*Non-comprehensive review of the relationship between tryptophan hydroxylase polymorphisms and personality traits/disorders in humans.*

## 4.2 Tryptophan in personality traits and disorders

The existing evidence regarding Trp interacting with personality and regulating trait-related behaviors has been reviewed and presented in **Table 2**. The acute tryptophan depletion (ATD) method has been developed to reduce plasma and

| Factor | Sample | Intervention | Effects on personality traits/ disorders | Ref. |
|---|---|---|---|---|
| Tryptophan condition | 52 male and female students | Acute Tryptophan Depletion (Young) | • Neuroticism discrimination is weakened | [47] |
| | 16 healthy males | Acute Tryptophan Depletion (Young) | • Discounting rates are increased in nine participants but are unchanged or decreased in seven participants<br>• Participants with increased discounting rate have higher neuroticism and lower self-directedness | [48] |
| | 28 healthy males | Tryptophan enhancement/ depletion | • Trait hostility and prolactin responses to tryptophan manipulation are negatively correlated following enhancement and positively following depletion | [49] |
| | 20 males with attention deficit hyperactivity disorder | Acute tryptophan depletion (Moja-De) | • Rates of reactive aggression in males with attention deficit hyperactivity disorder are decreased after low provocation | [50] |
| | 20 healthy males | | • Rates of reactive aggression in healthy males are increased after low provocation | |

| Factor | Sample | Intervention | Effects on personality traits/ disorders | Ref. |
|---|---|---|---|---|
| Tryptophan condition × Trait | 39 healthy males and 34 healthy females | Acute Tryptophan Depletion (Young) | • Guilt is preferentially elevated in highly empathic participants<br>• Annoyance is potentiated in participants high in trait psychopathy | [51] |
| | 24 high and 24 low trait aggression healthy males | Tryptophan enhancement/ depletion | • In aggressive traits, subjective and objective aggression is increased by tryptophan depletion and decreased by tryptophan enhancement<br>• Change in a low aggressive group is absent | [52] |
| | 13 young adults with and 12 without family history of mood disorder | Acute Tryptophan Depletion (Young) | • Abnormalities in emotional processing are detected in the individuals with no personal psychiatric history but at high familial risk for depression | [53] |
| | 22 male adolescents with attention deficit hyperactivity disorder | Acute tryptophan depletion (Moja-De) | • Aggressive behavior is increased in low-grade impulsive patients<br>• Aggressive behavior is not affected in high-grade impulsive patients | [54] |
| | 6 healthy subjects with high trait hostility and aggression and 6 with low | Acute tryptophan depletion (Moja-De) | • A rapid mood-lowering effect is detected on trait aggression healthy women<br>• No change is detected in high-aggressive men and low-aggressive women and men | [55] |
| | 34 low-hostile and 33 high-hostile individuals | Dietary tryptophan enhancement | • More negative mood and higher craving for alcohol are found in high-hostile individuals<br>• Subjective or physiological effects are not detected<br>• Stress-induced increase in craving is facilitated in high-hostile individuals by dietary tryptophan enhancement | [56] |

**Table 2.**
*Non-comprehensive review of the effects of tryptophan on personality traits and disorders in humans.*

cerebrospinal fluid Trp availability and central 5-HT concentrations, leading to alterations in personality and trait-related behaviors. Acute tryptophan depletion is firstly applied in humans by Concu et al. in 1977 [57]. And, the method has been modified by researchers, including Moja [58] and Young [59]. For example, the compositions of the amino acid mixtures are distinct [58, 59]. And, the gender difference is taken into account, i.e., the amino acid quantities of both ATD and placebo balanced beverages differ between males and females [47]. Moreover, inconsistencies exist regarding the effects of ATD on personality traits and disorders, attributing to the health state and characteristics of the subjects. For instance, ATD increases the rates of reactive aggression in healthy males, while it has opposite effect on males with ADHD [50]. Moreover, the trait property makes a difference. Guilt is preferentially elevated in highly empathic participants following ATD intervention, while annoyance is potentiated in participants high in trait psychopathy [51]. Hence, maternal plasma (MP) Trp fluctuation underlies the psychopathology of personality disorders, which may interfere fetal personality development via the maternal–fetal transmission, especially in the premise that personality already starts in the womb [3].

## 5. Maternal tryptophan fluctuation alters neuroendocrine and microbial development in offspring

Maternal Trp fluctuation induced by Trp-enriched or -depleted diets during pregnancy alters fetal neurogenesis and microbial constitution, which may reprogram the development and activity of the MGB, HPA, and HPG axes in offspring. The existing evidence has been reviewed and presented in **Table 3**.

The table is adjusted based on [10].

### 5.1 Maternal tryptophan fluctuation alters behavioral exhibition via reprogramming the neuroendocrine system in offspring

Maternal Trp fluctuation has altered the development and activity of the HPA axis in offspring indicated by the decreased plasma corticosterone (CORT) concentrations post restraint stress in the female adolescent mice experienced Trp-deficiency during the embryogenesis [73]. Low endogenous cortisol levels are associated with potentially pathological, intrusive, emotional memory processing [74, 75]. More specifically, the low posttraumatic urinary cortisol levels have been identified as a risk factor of posttraumatic stress disorder (PTSD) [74]. Moreover, maternal Trp administration in mice alters the development and function of the HPG axis during offspring's pubertal maturation via regulating the productions of prolactin (PRL) and luteinizing hormone (LH) in the pituitary gland [63, 65, 66]. Trp-free diets from gestation to puberty cause hypoandrogenism and hypoprolactinemia in the male progeny [65, 66], while maternal administration of Trp-enriched diets increases serum LH in offspring at postnatal (P) 70 days [63]. Increased serum PRL is associated with a diagnosis of BPD [76], and hyperprolactinemia has been observed in people with neurotic and personality disorders [77]. Moreover, a high serum PRL level is associated with psychological stress responses in humans [78]. An acute psychosocial stressor increases testosterone in both BPD patients and healthy participants [79].

### 5.2 Maternal tryptophan fluctuation alters behavioral exhibition via reprogramming the gut microbiota in offspring

Multi-hits early-life stress alters gut microbiome and brain gene expression, laying the foundation of mental health in postnatal life [80, 81]. The gut microbiota works

| Species | Treated Time | Control | Treatment | Exhibitions in offspring | Ref |
|---|---|---|---|---|---|
| Wistar rat | 14 days prior to mating–P4mo* | Standard chow powder (3.5 g tryptophan/kg) | 10 g tryptophan mixed with the diet (13.5 g tryptophan/kg) | • Decreased body weight of the male offspring at P4mo<br>• Decreased serotonin concentration, tryptophan hydroxylase 2 activity, and serotonin uptake in the frontal cortex and brain stem | [60] |
| Hypertensive rat | 7 continued days prior to mating | Stock chow diet | 30 mg ryptophan /kg/day mixed with the diet | • Increased body weight and blood pressure during P5wk–P15wk<br>• Increased brain weight at P20wk<br>• Increased total serotonin metabolite content in the medulla at P20wk | [61] |
| Sprague-Dawley rat | E17 | Saline vehicle | 200 mg tryptophan /kg oral gavage | • Increased tryptophan, serotonin, and 5-hydroxyindoleacetic acid concentrations in the fetal brain at E17 and E18 | [62] |
| Sprague-Dawley rat | E15–E21 | Saline vehicle | 200 mg tryptophan/kg oral gavage | • Increased serum prolactin at P40d and P70d<br>• Increased serum luteinizing hormone at P70d<br>• Increased forebrain serotonin and 5-hydroxyindoleacetic acid at P70d | [63] |
| Wistar rat | E19 and E21 | 0.1 N-HCl vehicle | 250 mg tryptophan /kg intraperitoneal | • Increased intracerebral concentrations of Trp at E19<br>• Decreased valine, methionine, leucine, tyrosine, phenylalanine, and histidine at E19<br>• Increased phosphoserine, threonine, serine, glutamic acid, and tryptophan at E21<br>• Decreased methionine, leucine, and histidine at E21<br>• Increased protein synthesis activity indicated by [$^3$H] Leucine incorporation at E19 and E21 | [64] |
| Sprague-Dawley rat | E14.5–late puberty | Control chow (0.22% tryptophan) | Tryptophan free diet (0.00% tryptophan) | • Dwarfism pups<br>• Decreased serum growth hormone concentration in male and female offspring<br>• Severe hypoprolactinemia<br>• Normal right-timed onset of puberty in both male and female rats | [65, 66] |

| Species | Treated Time | Control | Treatment | Exhibitions in offspring | Ref |
|---|---|---|---|---|---|
| Wistar rat | E5–E21 | Regular chow diet | Tryptophan-free diet (0.2% tryptophan) | • Unchanged brain weights in newborn pups<br>• Decreased body weight in newborn pups<br>• Reduced numbers of serotoninergic neurons at the dorsal raphe, especially at the medial and caudal sections of dorsal raphe, which contains the majority of serotoninergic neurons<br>• Unchanged brain serotonin concentration | [67] |
| Sprague-Dawley rat | E1–E21 | Control | 200 mg tryptophan/kg oral gavage | • Increased kidney weight-to-body weight ratio at P12wk<br>• Increase blood pressure in male offspring at P4wk, P6wk, P8wk, P10wk, and P12wk<br>• Decreased plasma level of L-citrulline (a precursor of L-arginine) and symmetric dimethylarginine (an indirect inhibitor of NO synthase)<br>• Increased mRNA expressions in the genes of aryl hydrocarbon receptor pathway | [68] |
| Chronic kidney disease Sprague-Dawley rat | E1–early postnatal life* | | | • Decreased systolic blood pressure, mean arterial pressure, and creatinine at P12wk<br>• Decreased plasma level of L-citrulline and symmetric dimethylarginine<br>• Altered the abundance of the tryptophan-metabolizing microbes, i.e., increased abundance of genus *Intestinimonas* and decreased abundance of genus *Turicibacter* | |
| Sprague-Dawley rat | E1–late puberty | Control chow (0.22% tryptophan) | Tryptophan free diet (0.00% tryptophan) | • Pronounced dwarfism pups<br>• Decreased serum growth hormone concentration in males and females<br>• Marked hypoandrogenism and severe hypoprolactinemia in males<br>• Hypoprolactinemia in females<br>• Right-timed pubertal maturation in both sexes | [65, 66] |

| Species | Treated Time | Control | Treatment | Exhibitions in offspring | Ref |
|---|---|---|---|---|---|
| Sprague-Dawley rat | E1–P12wk* | Control rat chow (0.22 g tryptophan p/100 g of pellets) | High- tryptophan diet (1 g tryptophan/100100 g of pellets) | • Increased blood serotonin, i.e., hyperserotonemia during P1wk–P12wk<br>• Decreased blood growth hormone<br>• Decreased activity of tryptophan hydroxylase1 in gastrointestinal tracts<br>• Decreased insulin-like growth factor-I expression in hepatic and muscle tissues | [69] |
| Sprague-Dawley rat | E1–weaning | 500 mg tryptophan /100 g diet | 75 mg tryptophan/100 g diet | • Decreased average body weight at weaning<br>• Unaffected opacities at P22d | [70] |
| Sprague-Dawley rat | E1–P25d * | TD.99366 control diet (1.8 g tryptophan /kg) | TD.08125 tryptophan-deficient diet (1 g tryptophan /kg) | • Normal body weight at P5d but reduced body weight at P15d and P25d<br>• Decreased body temperatures at P15d and P25d<br>• Unaffected oxygen consumption ($V_{O2}$)<br>• Altered breathing pattern and decreased heart rates at P15d<br>• Decreased ventilation ($V_E$) and $V_E$-to-$V_{O2}$ ratios in both air and 7% $CO_2$ at P25d<br>• Increased ventilatory response to $CO_2$ in male offspring at P5d and reduced at P15d and P25d in male and female offspring<br>• Reduced medullary serotonin concentration, while similar serotoninergic neuronal number | [71] |
| Pig | Third trimester of gestation–delivery | 2× tryptophan diet (0.26% tryptophan fed in the morning and afternoon) | High-low tryptophan diet (0.39% tryptophanfed in the morning and 0.13% tryptophan fed in the afternoon) | • Decreased birth healthy pig rate and birth weight of piglet per pen with similar total birth weight per pen<br>• Decreased serum phosphoserine, taurine, cysteine, proline in newborns and increased liver *n*-6:*n*-3 polyunsaturated fat ratio<br>• Altered gene expressions, including the genes related to cytotoxic effector regulation, nicotinamide adenine dinucleotide oxidation, reactive oxygen species metabolism, and tissue development | [72] |

| Species | Treated Time | Control | Treatment | Exhibitions in offspring | Ref |
|---|---|---|---|---|---|
| Outbred CD-1 mouse | Lactation (P0d–P8d) | Standard laboratory diet (0.14% tryptophan) | Tryptophan-deficient diet (0.00% tryptophan) | • Unchanged time spent in open sectors in the 0-maze test in adolescent daughters (P189d–P193d)<br>• Unchanged time spent in floating in the forced-swim test in adolescent daughters<br>• Unchanged time spent in the novel compartment in the novelty-seeking test in adolescent daughters<br>• Unchanged achieved breakpoint in the progressive ratio operant procedure in adolescent daughters<br>• Decreased plasma corticosterone concentrations and similar brain-derived neurotrophic factor concentrations following restraint stress in adolescent daughters | [73] |

**The pups are fed the same diet as mothers throughout postnatal (P) life.*

**Table 3.**
*Non-comprehensive review of the effects of maternal tryptophan administration on offspring behavioral and physiological exhibitions in experimental animals.*

as a virtual endocrine organ [82]. It has been demonstrated in the chronic kidney disease (CKD) rats that gestational Trp prevents hypertension via reprograming the Trp-metabolic microbiome in offspring, increasing the abundance of genus *Intestinimonas* and decreasing the abundance of genus *Turicibacter* [68]. The abundance of *Turicibacter* is negatively associated with sociability traits [83]. Moreover, gut microbes regulate stress responses, i.e., the activity of the HPA axis, via the MGB axis. A decreased abundance of *Lactobacillus* has been associated with increased stress reactivity in the infant rhesus monkeys that experienced maternal separation [84].

### 5.3 The accompanied physiological alterations are associated with the neuropsychological impairment in offspring

The physiological alterations in the offspring following the maternal Trp administration, such as the changes in body weight (BW), blood pressure, and breath movement [60, 61, 65–68, 70–72, 85], may be underlying the altered neuroendocrine and gut microbial development. For example, host's eating behavior is manipulated by the gut microbes and neuroendocrine cells [86], which determines the growth of BW. The National Collaborative Perinatal Project (NCPP, New England) revealed a relationship between obstetrical complications and neuropsychological deficits in children aged 7 [87]. The dissatisfaction with body image followed by improper Trp administrations may have counterbalanced mental health, causing negative influences on the psychosocial development in offspring.

## 6. Inconsistency and barriers

### 6.1 Inconsistency in maternal tryptophan programming offspring neuropsychiatric development

This is not surprising that the outcomes of prenatal Trp exposure are of complex phenotypes, due to a sequential series of events during embryogenesis. Taking as an example the central nervous system (CNS), a sensitive target for gestational Trp exposure experiences vast majority of differentiation at cellular and nucleus levels. A small or subtle alteration in brain structure during fetal development can be progressively magnified over time and moderated by postnatal conditions, affecting emotional regulation and decision-making [88]. Issues are likely to cause inconsistency in the current findings, including the pregnancy stage of Trp taken, its intensity, and pregnant women's age, eating habits, lifestyle, and health status. For example, in Wistar rats, the brain 5-HT concentration, TPH2 activity, and 5-HT uptake in offspring are decreased by fed a 10 g Trp-enriched diet from 2 weeks prior to mating through postnatal life [60] while administrated 30 mg/kg/day of Trp mixed with a stock chow diet for 1 week prior to mating increases total 5-HT metabolite content in the medulla at P20wk in the offspring of hypertensive rats [61]. Moreover, plasma Trp concentrations vary across maternal seasonality and season of conception [89]. Hence, the influence of the environment and other exogenous agents should be considered when studying the causality between maternal Trp fluctuation and neuropsychiatric development in offspring. The longitudinal studies of gestational Trp impacts are also advocated, because the early-life adversity can be masked by favorable experiences at a later age, such as family support, culture, and education [17].

### 6.2 The microbial barrier for investigating the fetal exposure on neuropsychiatric development

The maternal-fetal microbe transmission during pregnancy, vaginal delivery, and breastfeeding constitutes the initial gut microbiome in the progeny of humans and other viviparous mammals. Given the comorbid gastrointestinal symptoms of neurodevelopmental disorders [20], prenatal stimuli altering neurogenesis may have perturbed maternal-fetal microbe transmission and altered the gut microbiome and MGB axis functioning in the progeny [80, 81]. However, early-life predisposition can be buffered or masked by the postnatal life experience [17]. Hence, the later-life events, such as eating, diseases, medicine, may interrupt the offspring gut microbial development and veil the early-life effect on the MGB axis, as a barrier in the investigation of fetal exposure altering neuropsychiatric development [90].

### 6.3 Ethical issues in human and rodent research

Maternal Trp fluctuation potentially alters fetal brain and gastrointestinal development. However, it is not possible to determine fetal changes for logistical and ethical reasons in humans. Aborted fetuses from women undergoing pregnancy termination have been recruited to determine the neuroendocrinological alterations caused by maternal diseases or over-the-counter (OTC) and prescription drug administrations during pregnancy worldwide since 1973 [91]. However, a survey in 2012 revealed the fact that this kind of research is not likely to be approved by most North American medical institutions for ethical considerations [92]. Moreover, assessing fetal exposure effect is limited to a single cord plasma concentration measured at the time of delivery, i.e., real-time monitoring of fetal neuroendocrine profile is not allowed. However, in most clinical cases, the ratio of umbilical vein (UV) to maternal plasma (MP) does not reflect the exact fetal drug exposure relative to mother [93].

Rodents are widely used in preclinical pharmacologic research in assessing fetal exposure and investigating the underlying mechanisms, but the outcomes of experimental animal models have difficulty in extrapolating to clinical decisions. In viviparous animals, the variable litter size and gestational age cannot be accurately predicted; a great number of matings are needed to meet a certain sample size for sufficient statistical power; the female parent per se must be euthanized for sampling [90]. These go against the 3Rs of animal ethics, which advocate to minimize invasiveness, restrict animals subjected to potentially harmful procedures, and cut down the number of animals sacrificed, i.e., Replacement, Reduction, and Refinement [94].

## 7. Thinking chicken

### 7.1 Chicken embryo model

The advantages and disadvantages of human, rodent, and chicken models in investigating ontogenetic origin of neuropsychiatric disorders have been summarized in **Table 4**. The chicken embryo is a mainstay model for safety assessment in maternal-fetal medicine and mechanistic study due to its special biological characteristics: high reproducibility, time- and cost-saving preparation, self-contained development, precise litter size, accessibility, and easy in vivo experimental manipulation [95].

| Species | Human | Rodent | Chicken |
|---|---|---|---|
| Advantages | • Closed to the clinical decisions<br>• Equipped with placenta | • Accessibility<br>• Approachable prenatal development<br>• Equipped with placenta<br>• Developing modern mechanistic approaches have been applied<br>• Genetically engineered mouse models available | • Accessibility<br>• Time- and cost-saving<br>• High reproducibility providing sufficient sample size for statistical power<br>• Precise litter size<br>• Accurate developmental stages<br>• Large embryos with a uniform genetic background<br>• Easy in vivo experimental manipulation with the availability of a number of techniques<br>• Self-sustained development |
| Disadvantages | • Ethical issues<br>• Maternal metabolism influence<br>• Maternal microbe transfer<br>• Single time-point detection | • Sacrifice of the female parent<br>• Unprecise and small litter size<br>• Small embryos<br>• Hard to predict the embryonic stage<br>• Maternal metabolism influence<br>• Maternal microbe transfer<br>• Time-consuming and high cost | • Lack of placenta<br>• Lack of developing modern mechanistic approaches<br>• Lack of genetically engineered models |

*The table is adjusted based on [90].*

**Table 4.**
*A comparative summary among human, rodent, and chicken models in investigating ontogenetic origin of neuropsychiatric disorders.*

Moreover, in viviparous animals, the placenta mediates the nutrient transfer between maternal and embryonic circulations [96]. The closed system prolongs chicken embryonic exposure to xenobiotics without excretion until hatching, reducing the stress caused by multiple injections in determining the toxic influence on fetal development and subsequent neuroendocrine alterations [97].

## 7.2 Chicken embryo for studying ontogenetic origin of neuropsychiatric disorders

As a sensitive target, heterogeneity exists in diverse brain regions at various embryonic stages, which is crucial for investigating ontogenetic origin of neuropsychiatric disorders, i.e., a dynamic and comprehensive perspective. In maternal-fetal medicine, the drug candidates need to be vigorously assessed using toxicological, pharmacokinetic, and pharmacological tests as well as electrophysiological, neurophysiological, and behavioral measures before clinical trials can begin. The chicken embryo model has been widely employed to investigate fetal neuropathology post antiepileptic exposure [95] as well as to determine neurotoxic effects of steroid hormones on the immature cerebellum [98].

Before hatching, the embryonic experience and genetic determinants have cooperated in developing postnatal cognition and behavior, which makes chickens central to understanding the interface between predisposition and experience-based learning at the beginning of life [99, 100]. A chick exhibits behavioral responses shortly after hatching via inherited predisposed and learning mechanisms, which shapes cognition [100]. Moreover, the large size of the chicken embryo and self-sustained embryonic development allow easy in vivo manipulation. The neurobiological basis underlying early social predispositions is being uncovered in chickens, and functional similarities have been identified between the brains of chickens and mammals [101]. For example, the avian forebrain is derived from the same anatomical substrate as mammals, demonstrating the cognitive similarity across species [102]. Hence, the chicken embryo offers a trustworthy and suitable model for investigating ontogenetic origin of neuropsychiatric disorders.

### 7.3 Embryonic serotonin exposure reduces aggression while embryonic tryptophan exposure yields bullying victims

The 5-HT and dopamine (DA) systems interact at a basic neurophysiological level in regulating impulsive aggression, which plays a critical role in several mental disorders, including BPD and antisocial personality disorder [103]. Similar to it in humans, aggression in chickens is related to personality disorders [104]. In ovo 5-HT injection (10 μg/egg) reduces aggressive behaviors at a cost of increased fearfulness during adolescence and before sex maturation in the White Leghorn chickens [105]. The results in the Dekalb XL birds, a highly aggressive strain [106, 107], indicate that prenatal 5-HT exposure (10 and 20 μg/egg) reduces aggression via regulating the 5-HT availability or DA storage and reprogramming the development of the HPA axis [11].

Bullying involvement is related to personality development [108]. Gut microbiota has a measurable impact on social performance via mediating the MGB axis; in turn, social interactions are involved in shaping the gut microbial community [109]. In a study, Trp administration (500 μg/egg) in White Leghorn chickens at E12 yields bullying victims, indicated by reduced body weight and aggressive behaviors in the male offspring before and during adolescence, attributing to the altered function of the MGB and HPA axes [12]. Briefly, the intestinal histomorphology has been altered in the Trp-treated roosters, i.e., the increased crypt depth and decreased villus/crypt ratio in the ileum-jejunum junction, indicating an altered gut microenvironment and reduced surface for absorbing nutrients. Corresponding changes in the cecal microbiota composition, i.e., the increased abundances of genera *Ruminococcaceae UCG-005*, *Olsenella*, *Ruminococcus_2*, and *Oscillospira*, have been identified in the Trp-treated roosters [12], which are the core microbes in human colonic crypt [110]. In this way, a low abundance of genus *Oscillospira* has been characterized in aggressive dogs compared with normal behavior group [111]. Moreover, a high abundance of genus *Olsenella* has been associated with low BW in the Japanese population and observed in female MDD patients [112, 113]. In the trier social stress test (TSST), peer victimization exhibits more stress with an altered HPA axis activity [114]. The HPA axis is developmentally cross-linked with the gut microbiota [115], which hints the gut microbes' role in neurogenesis and behavioral development in offspring. Hence, the increased catecholamine concentrations in the chicken hypothalamus post embryonic Trp exposure indicate an altered HPA axis activity and may be associated with the altered gut microbiome and MGB axis function, mediating impulsive aggression confronting conflictual peer interactions [90].

## 8. Conclusions

This chapter discusses the relationship of TPH polymorphisms and Trp administrations with personality traits/disorders, which bridges the Trp metabolism in pregnant women and neuropsychiatric disorders in offspring. Gestational Trp participates in the development of the CNS and gastrointestinal system, which reciprocally interact via the MGB axis, shaping long-standing patterns of cognition and behavior. The chicken embryo can be a good model for investigating maternal effects on offspring neuropsychiatric development due to that it skirts the maternal influences on the neuroendocrine and gastrointestinal development, i.e., maternal metabolic fluctuation and maternal-fetal microbe transmission seen in humans and other mammals. Moreover, the behavioral response can be tested shortly after hatching due to social predispositions in chickens, which can be intervened during embryogenesis. Accumulated evidence in chicken embryonic development indicates that embryonic exposures to Trp and its metabolite, 5-HT, reprogram neuroendocrine and MGB axis in offspring, attenuating aggression and defeated in bullying. Herein, maintaining an appropriate Trp level by controlling dietary Trp and rigorous medication therapy during pregnancy has been advocated as a biotherapeutic targeting strategy for preventing personality disorders and comorbid psychosocial dysfunctions.

## Author details

Xiaohong Huang[1,2*], Xiaohua Li[3] and Heng-Wei Cheng[2,4]

1 Department of Sports Medicine, The Affiliated Hospital of Qingdao University, Qingdao, Shandong, China

2 Department of Animal Sciences, Purdue University, West Lafayette, IN, USA

3 School of Basic Medical Sciences, Qingdao University, Qingdao, Shandong, China

4 Livestock Behavior Research Unit, USDA-ARS, West Lafayette, IN, USA

*Address all correspondence to: ysrred@gmail.com

## References

[1] Asselmann E et al. The role of personality in the thoughts, feelings, and behaviors of students in Germany during the first weeks of the COVID-19 pandemic. PloS One. 2020;**15**(11):e0242904. DOI: 10.1371/journal.pone.0242904

[2] Björkenstam E et al. Association between childhood adversity and a diagnosis of personality disorder in young adulthood: a cohort study of 107,287 individuals in Stockholm County. European Journal of Epidemiology. 2017;**32**(8):721-731. DOI: 10.1007/s10654-017-0264-9

[3] Gartstein M, Skinner M. Prenatal influences on temperament development: the role of environmental epigenetics. Development and Psychopathology. 2018;**30**(4):1269-1303. DOI: 10.1017/s0954579417001730

[4] Brannigan R et al. The role of prenatal stress as a pathway to personality disorder: longitudinal birth cohort study. The British journal of Psychiatry: The Journal of Mental Science. 2020;**216**(2):85-89. DOI: 10.1192/bjp.2019.190

[5] Cackowski S et al. Anger and aggression in borderline personality disorder and attention deficit hyperactivity disorder - does stress matter? Borderline Personality Disorder and Emotion Dysregulation. 2017;**4**:6. DOI: 10.1186/s40479-017-0057-5

[6] Wilson ST et al. The tryptophan hydroxylase-1 A218C polymorphism is associated with diagnosis, but not suicidal behavior, in borderline personality disorder. American Journal of Medical Genetics Part B: Neuropsychiatric Genetics. 2009;**150**(2):202-208. DOI: 10.1002/ajmg.b.30788

[7] Zaboli G et al. Tryptophan hydroxylase-1 gene variants associate with a group of suicidal borderline women. Neuropsychopharmacology. 2006;**31**(9):1982-1990. DOI: 10.1038/sj.npp.1301046

[8] Perez-Rodriguez MM et al. Tryptophan-hydroxylase 2 haplotype association with borderline personality disorder and aggression in a sample of patients with personality disorders and healthy controls. Journal of Psychiatric Research. 2010;**44**(15):1075-1081. DOI: 10.1016/j.jpsychires.2010.03.014

[9] Badawy AA-B. Tryptophan metabolism, disposition and utilization in pregnancy. Bioscience Reports. 2015;**35**(5):e00261. DOI: 10.1042/bsr20150197

[10] Huang X, Feng Z, Cheng H-w. Perspective: gestational tryptophan fluctuation altering neuroembryogenesis and psychosocial development. Cells. 2022;**11**(8):1270. DOI: 10.3390/cells11081270

[11] Huang X et al. Prenatal serotonin fluctuation affects serotoninergic development and related neural circuits in chicken embryos. Neuroscience. 2021;**473**:66-80. DOI: 10.1016/j.neuroscience.2021.08.011

[12] Huang X et al. Embryonic exposure to tryptophan yields bullying victimization via reprogramming the microbiota-gut-brain axis in a chicken model. Nutrients. 2022;**14**(3):661. DOI: 10.3390/nu14030661

[13] Kerekes N et al. ADHD, autism spectrum disorder, temperament, and character: phenotypical associations and etiology in a Swedish childhood

twin study. Comprehensive Psychiatry. 2013;**54**(8):1140-1147. DOI: 10.1016/j.comppsych.2013.05.009

[14] Rausch J et al. Associations between age and cortisol awakening response in patients with borderline personality disorder. Journal of Neural Transmission. 2021;**128**(9):1425-1432. DOI: 10.1007/s00702-021-02402-3

[15] Carrasco J et al. Hypothalamic-pituitary-adrenal axis response in borderline personality disorder without post-traumatic features. The British Journal of Psychiatry. 2007;**190**:357-358. DOI: 10.1192/bjp.bp.106.022590

[16] Tackett J et al. Personality × hormone interactions in adolescent externalizing psychopathology. Personality Disorders. 2014;**5**(3):235-246. DOI: 10.1037/per0000075

[17] Barker DJ. The fetal origins of adult disease. Fetal and Maternal Medicine Review. 1994;**6**(2):71-80. DOI: 10.1017/S0965539500001005

[18] Montgomery, A.K., et al., Maternal serotonin levels are associated with cognitive ability and core symptoms in autism spectrum disorder. Journal of the American Academy of Child & Adolescent Psychiatry, 2018. **57**(11): p. 867-875, doi: 10.1016/j.jaac.2018.06.025.

[19] Coste J et al. Risk of early neurodevelopmental disorders associated with in utero exposure to valproate and other antiepileptic drugs: a nationwide cohort study in France. Scientific Reports. 2020;**10**(1):17362. DOI: 10.1038/s41598-020-74409-x

[20] Kim J-W et al. Gastrointestinal tract abnormalities induced by prenatal valproic acid exposure in rat offspring. Toxicological Research. 2013;**29**(3):173-179. DOI: 10.5487/TR.2013.29.3.173

[21] De Angelis M et al. Fecal microbiota and metabolome of children with autism and pervasive developmental disorder not otherwise specified. PloS One. 2013;**8**(10):e76993. DOI: 10.1371/journal.pone.0076993

[22] Bonnin A et al. A transient placental source of serotonin for the fetal forebrain. Nature. 2011;**472**(7343):347-350. DOI: 10.1038/nature09972

[23] Bonnin A et al. Serotonin modulates the response of embryonic thalamocortical axons to netrin-1. Nature Neuroscience. 2007;**10**(5):588-597. DOI: 10.1038/nn1896

[24] Joyce P et al. The presence of both serotonin 1A receptor (HTR1A) and dopamine transporter (DAT1) gene variants increase the risk of borderline personality disorder. Frontiers in Genetics. 2014;**4**:313. DOI: 10.3389/fgene.2013.00313

[25] Karahoda R et al. Dynamics of tryptophan metabolic pathways in human placenta and placental-derived cells: effect of gestation age and trophoblast differentiation. Frontiers in Cell and Developmental Biology. 2020;**8**:574034. DOI: 10.3389/fcell.2020.574034

[26] Anderson G, Maes M. Schizophrenia: linking prenatal infection to cytokines, the tryptophan catabolite (TRYCAT) pathway, NMDA receptor hypofunction, neurodevelopment and neuroprogression. Progress in Neuro-Psychopharmacology and Biological Psychiatry. 2013;**42**:5-19. DOI: 10.1016/j.pnpbp.2012.06.014

[27] Keane JM et al. Identifying a biological signature of prenatal maternal stress. JCI Insight. 2021;**6**(2):e143007. DOI: 10.1172/jci.insight.143007

[28] Tenhola S et al. Blood pressure, serum lipids, fasting insulin, and adrenal

hormones in 12-year-old children born with maternal preeclampsia. The Journal of Clinical Endocrinology and Metabolism. 2003;**88**(3):1217-1222. DOI: 10.1210/jc.2002-020903

[29] Sun B et al. Association of preeclampsia in term births with neurodevelopmental disorders in offspring. JAMA Psychiatry. 2020;**77**(8):823-829. DOI: 10.1001/jamapsychiatry.2020.0306

[30] Law K et al. Tryptophan and purine metabolites are consistently upregulated in the urinary metabolome of patients diagnosed with gestational diabetes mellitus throughout pregnancy: a longitudinal metabolomics study of Chinese pregnant women part 2. Clinica Chimica Acta; International Journal of Clinical Chemistry. 2017;**468**:126-139. DOI: 10.1016/j.cca.2017.02.018

[31] Rowland J, Wilson C. The association between gestational diabetes and ASD and ADHD: a systematic review and meta-analysis. Scientific Reports. 2021;**11**(1):5136. DOI: 10.1038/s41598-021-84573-3

[32] Notarangelo FM, Schwarcz R. Restraint stress during pregnancy rapidly raises kynurenic acid levels in mouse placenta and fetal brain. Developmental Neuroscience. 2016;**38**(6):458-468. DOI: 10.1159/000455228

[33] Galley JD et al. Prenatal stress-induced disruptions in microbial and host tryptophan metabolism and transport. Behavioural Brain Research. 2021;**414**:113471. DOI: 10.1016/j.bbr.2021.113471

[34] Kim S et al. The effects of serotonin transporter promoter and monoamine oxidase A gene polymorphisms on trait emotional intelligence. Neuropsychobiology. 2011;**64**(4):224-230. DOI: 10.1159/000327705

[35] Manuck S et al. Aggression and anger-related traits associated with a polymorphism of the tryptophan hydroxylase gene. Biological Psychiatry. 1999;**45**(5):603-614. DOI: 10.1016/s0006-3223(98)00375-8

[36] Baud P et al. Modulation of anger control in suicide attempters by TPH-1. Genes, Brain, and Behavior. 2009;**8**(1):97-100. DOI: 10.1111/j.1601-183X.2008.00451.x

[37] Suzuki A et al. No association between the TPH A218C polymorphism and personality traits in Japanese healthy subjects. Progress in Neuro-Psychopharmacology & Biological Psychiatry. 2007;**31**(2):395-398. DOI: 10.1016/j.pnpbp.2006.10.003

[38] Yang J et al. Association between tryptophan hydroxylase 2 polymorphism and anger-related personality traits among young Korean women. Neuropsychobiology. 2010;**62**(3):158-163. DOI: 10.1159/000318572

[39] Cuartas Arias J et al. Exploring epistasis in candidate genes for antisocial personality disorder. Psychiatric Genetics. 2011;**21**(3):115-124. DOI: 10.1097/YPG.0b013e3283437175

[40] Rujescu D et al. Association of anger-related traits with SNPs in the TPH gene. Molecular Psychiatry. 2002;7(9):1023-1029. DOI: 10.1038/sj.mp.4001128

[41] Reuter M, Hennig J. Pleiotropic effect of the TPH A779C polymorphism on nicotine dependence and personality. American Journal of Medical Genetics. Part B, Neuropsychiatric Genetics. 2005;**134**(1):20-24. DOI: 10.1002/ajmg.b.30153

[42] Tochigi M et al. No association of 5-HT2C, 5-HT6, and tryptophan hydroxylase-1 gene polymorphisms

with personality traits in the Japanese population. Neuroscience Letters. 2006;**403**:100-102. DOI: 10.1016/j.neulet.2006.04.020

[43] Laas K et al. Nice guys: homozygocity for the TPH2-703G/T (rs4570625) minor allele promotes low aggressiveness and low anxiety. Journal of Affective Disorders. 2017;**215**:230-236. DOI: 10.1016/j.jad.2017.03.045

[44] Lehto K et al. Effect of tryptophan hydroxylase-2 gene polymorphism G-703 T on personality in a population representative sample. Progress in Neuro-Psychopharmacology and Biological Psychiatry. 2015;**57**:31-35. DOI: 10.1016/j.pnpbp.2014.10.005

[45] Yoon H et al. Impact of tryptophan hydroxylase 2 G-703T polymorphism on anger-related personality traits and orbitofrontal cortex. Behavioural Brain Research. 2012;**231**(1):105-110. DOI: 10.1016/j.bbr.2012.03.001

[46] Gutknecht L et al. Tryptophan hydroxylase-2 gene variation influences personality traits and disorders related to emotional dysregulation. The International Journal of Neuropsychopharmacology. 2007;**10**(3):309-320. DOI: 10.1017/s1461145706007437

[47] Ward R et al. The role of serotonin in personality inference: tryptophan depletion impairs the identification of neuroticism in the face. Psychopharmacology. 2017;**234**(14):2139-2147

[48] Demoto Y et al. Neural and personality correlates of individual differences related to the effects of acute tryptophan depletion on future reward evaluation. Neuropsychobiology. 2012;**65**(2):55-64. DOI: 10.1159/000328990

[49] Wingrove J et al. Trait hostility and prolactin response to tryptophan enhancement/depletion. Neuropsychobiology. 1999;**40**(4):202-206. DOI: 10.1159/000026620

[50] Zimmermann M et al. The effects of acute tryptophan depletion on reactive aggression in adults with attention-deficit/hyperactivity disorder (ADHD) and healthy controls. PloS One. 2012;**7**(3):e32023. DOI: 10.1371/journal.pone.0032023

[51] Kanen JW et al. Serotonin depletion amplifies distinct human social emotions as a function of individual differences in personality. Translational Psychiatry. 2021;**11**(1):1-12. DOI: 10.1038/s41398-020-00880-9

[52] Cleare A, Bond A. The effect of tryptophan depletion and enhancement on subjective and behavioural aggression in normal male subjects. Psychopharmacology. 1995;**118**(1):72-81. DOI: 10.1007/BF02245252

[53] Feder A et al. Tryptophan depletion and emotional processing in healthy volunteers at high risk for depression. Biological Psychiatry. 2011;**69**(8):804-807. DOI: 10.1016/j.biopsych.2010.12.033

[54] Zepf F et al. Serotonergic functioning and trait-impulsivity in attention-deficit/hyperactivity-disordered boys (ADHD): influence of rapid tryptophan depletion. Human Psychopharmacology. 2008;**23**(1):43-51. DOI: 10.1002/hup.896

[55] Schmeck K et al. Mood changes following acute tryptophan depletion in healthy adults. Psychopathology. 2002;**35**(4):234-240. DOI: 10.1159/000063827

[56] Nesic J, Duka T. Effects of stress on emotional reactivity in hostile

heavy social drinkers following dietary tryptophan enhancement. Alcohol & Alcoholism. 2008;**43**(2):151-162. DOI: 10.1093/alcalc/agm179

[57] Concu A et al. Mental changes induced by the oral administration of tryptophan-free amino acid mixtures in man. IRCS Medical Science. 1977;**5**:520

[58] Moja E et al. Increase in stage 4 sleep after ingestion of a tryptophan-free diet in humans. Pharmacological Research Communications. 1984;**16**(9):909-914. DOI: 10.1016/s0031-6989(84)80027-2

[59] Young SN et al. Tryptophan depletion causes a rapid lowering of mood in normal males. Psychopharmacology. 1985;**87**(2):173-177. DOI: 10.1007/BF00431803

[60] Huether G, Thömke F, Adler L. Administration of tryptophan-enriched diets to pregnant rats retards the development of the serotonergic system in their offspring. Developmental Brain Research. 1992;**68**(2):175-181. DOI: 10.1016/0165-3806(92)90059-6

[61] Ito H et al. Effects of tryptophane on SHRSP offspring growth. Clinical and Experimental Hypertension. Part A: Theory and Practice. 1991;**13**(5):971-979. DOI: 10.3109/10641969109042103

[62] Arevalo R et al. Fetal brain serotonin synthesis and catabolism is under control by mother intake of tryptophan. Life Sciences. 1991;**49**(1):53-66. DOI: 10.1016/0024-3205(91)90579-z

[63] Martin L et al. Tryptophan ingestion by gestant mothers alters prolactin and luteinizing hormone release in the adult male offspring. Brain Research. 1997;**774**(1-2):265-268. DOI: 10.1016/s0006-8993(97)81718-0

[64] Fando JL, Domínguez F, Herrera E. Tryptophan overload in the pregnant rat: effect on brain amino acid levels and in vitro protein synthesis. Journal of Neurochemistry. 1981;**37**(4):824-829. DOI: 10.1111/j.1471-4159.1981.tb04467.x

[65] Imbesi R, Castrogiovanni P. Embryonic and postnatal development in experimental tryptophan deprived rats. A preliminary study. Journal of Molecular Histology. 2008;**39**(5):487-498. DOI: 10.1007/s10735-008-9188-8

[66] Imbesi R, Mazzone V, Castrogiovanni P. Is tryptophan 'more'essential than other essential aminoacids in development? A morphologic study. Anatomia, Histologia, Embryologia. 2009;**38**(5):361-369. DOI: 10.1111/j.1439-0264.2009.00955.x

[67] Flores-Cruz GM, Escobar A. Reduction of serotonergic neurons in the dorsal raphe due to chronic prenatal administration of a tryptophan-free diet. International Journal of Developmental Neuroscience. 2012;**30**(2):63-67. DOI: 10.1016/j.ijdevneu.2012.01.002

[68] Hsu C-N et al. Maternal tryptophan supplementation protects adult rat offspring against hypertension programmed by maternal chronic kidney disease: implication of tryptophan-metabolizing microbiome and aryl hydrocarbon receptor. International Journal of Molecular Sciences. 2020;**21**(12):4552. DOI: 10.3390/ijms21124552

[69] Castrogiovanni P et al. Effects of high-tryptophan diet on pre-and postnatal development in rats: a morphological study. European Journal of Nutrition. 2014;**53**(1):297-308. DOI: 10.1007/s00394-013-0528-4

[70] Bunce GE, Hess JL. Lenticular opacities in young rats as a consequence of maternal diets low in tryptophan and/

or vitamin E. The Journal of Nutrition. 1976;**106**(2):222-229. DOI: 10.1093/jn/106.2.222

[71] Penatti EM et al. Maternal dietary tryptophan deficiency alters cardiorespiratory control in rat pups. Journal of Applied Physiology. 2011;**110**(2):318-328. DOI: 10.1152/japplphysiol.00788.2010

[72] Xu K et al. Negative effects on newborn piglets caused by excess dietary tryptophan in the morning in sows. Journal of the Science of Food and Agriculture. 2019;**99**(6):3005-3016. DOI: 10.1002/jsfa.9514

[73] Zoratto F et al. Effects of maternal L-tryptophan depletion and corticosterone administration on neurobehavioral adjustments in mouse dams and their adolescent and adult daughters. Progress in Neuro-Psychopharmacology and Biological Psychiatry. 2011;**35**(6):1479-1492. DOI: 10.1016/j.pnpbp.2011.02.016

[74] Delahanty D, Raimonde A, Spoonster E. Initial posttraumatic urinary cortisol levels predict subsequent PTSD symptoms in motor vehicle accident victims. Biological Psychiatry. 2000;**48**(9):940-947. DOI: 10.1016/s0006-3223(00)00896-9

[75] Wirth M et al. The effect of cortisol on emotional responses depends on order of cortisol and placebo administration in a within-subject design. Psychoneuroendocrinology. 2011;**36**(7):945-954. DOI: 10.1016/j.psyneuen.2010.11.010

[76] Atmaca M et al. Increased serum prolactin in borderline personality disorder. The International Journal of Psychiatry in Medicine. 2015;**49**(3):169-175. DOI: 10.1177/0091217415582172

[77] Rutkowski K et al. Hyper-prolactinemia phenomenon in neurotic and personality disorders and changes in prolactin level after the psychotherapy. European Psychiatry. 2017;**41**(S1):S260-S260. DOI: 10.1016/j.eurpsy.2017.02.067

[78] Lennartsson A-K, Jonsdottir IH. Prolactin in response to acute psychosocial stress in healthy men and women. Psychoneuroendocrinology. 2011;**36**(10):1530-1539. DOI: 10.1016/j.psyneuen.2011.04.007

[79] Deuter C et al. Psychosocial stress increases testosterone in patients with borderline personality disorder, post-traumatic stress disorder and healthy participants. Borderline Personality Disorder and Emotion Dysregulation. 2021;**8**(1):3. DOI: 10.1186/s40479-021-00145-x

[80] Usui N, Matsuzaki H, Shimada S. Characterization of early life stress-affected gut microbiota. Brain Sciences. 2021;**11**(7):913. DOI: 10.3390/brainsci11070913

[81] Rincel M et al. Multi-hit early life adversity affects gut microbiota, brain and behavior in a sex-dependent manner. Brain, Behavior, and Immunity. 2019;**80**:179-192. DOI: 10.1016/j.bbi.2019.03.006

[82] Cheng H-w, Jiang S, Hu J. Gut-brain axis: probiotic, *Bacillus subtilis*, prevents aggression via the modification of the central serotonergic system. In: Mahmoudi R, Moosazad S, Aghaei K, editors. Oral Health by Using Probiotic Products. London, UK: IntechOpen; 2019

[83] Szyszkowicz JK et al. Implications of the gut microbiota in vulnerability to the social avoidance effects of chronic social defeat in male mice. Brain, Behavior, and

Immunity. 2017;**66**:45-55. DOI: 10.1016/j.bbi.2017.06.009

[84] Bailey MT, Coe CL. Maternal separation disrupts the integrity of the intestinal microflora in infant rhesus monkeys. Developmental Psychobiology. 1999;**35**(2):146-155

[85] Devoe LD et al. Maternal dietary substrates and human fetal biophysical activity: I. The effects of tryptophan and glucose on fetal breathing movements. American Journal of Obstetrics and Gynecology. 1986;**155**(1):135-139. DOI: 10.1016/0002-9378(86)90096-7

[86] Farzi A, Fröhlich E, Holzer P. Gut microbiota and the neuroendocrine system. Neurotherapeutics. 2018;**15**(1):5-22. DOI: 10.1007/s13311-017-0600-5

[87] Seidman LJ et al. The relationship of prenatal and perinatal complications to cognitive functioning at age 7 in the New England Cohorts of the National Collaborative Perinatal Project. Schizophrenia Bulletin. 2000;**26**(2):309-321. DOI: 10.1093/oxfordjournals.schbul.a033455

[88] Entringer S. Prenatal stress exposure and fetal programming of complex phenotypes: interactive effects with multiple risk factors. Neuroscience and Biobehavioral Reviews. 2020;**117**:3-4. DOI: 10.1016/j.neubiorev.2020.04.002

[89] Levitan RD et al. Seasonality of plasma tryptophan and kynurenine in pregnant mothers with a history of seasonal affective disorder: vulnerability or adaptation? The World Journal of Biological Psychiatry. 2020;**21**(7):529-538. DOI: 10.1080/15622975.2020.1769189

[90] Huang X, Cheng H-w. Perspective: chicken models for studying the ontogenetic origin of neuropsychiatric disorders. Biomedicines. 2022;**10**(5):1115. DOI: 10.3390/biomedicines10051155

[91] Cates W, Grimes DA, Schulz KF. The public health impact of legal abortion: 30 years later. Perspectives on Sexual and Reproductive Health. 2003;**35**(1):25-28. DOI: 10.1363/3502503

[92] Gedeon C, Nava-Ocampo AA, Koren G. Ethical issues in pharmacologic research in women undergoing pregnancy termination: a systemic review and survey of researchers. Obstetrics and Gynecology International. 2012;**2012**:724591. DOI: 10.1155/2012/724591

[93] Zhang Z et al. Development of a novel maternal-fetal physiologically based pharmacokinetic model I: insights into factors that determine fetal drug exposure through simulations and sensitivity analyses. Drug Metabolism and Disposition. 2017;**45**(8):920-938. DOI: 10.1124/dmd.117.075192

[94] Cheluvappa R, Scowen P, Eri R. Ethics of animal research in human disease remediation, its institutional teaching; and alternatives to animal experimentation. Pharmacology Research & Perspectives. 2017;**5**(4):e00332. DOI: 10.1002/prp2.332

[95] Zosen D et al. Chicken embryo as animal model to study drug distribution to the developing brain. Journal of Pharmacological and Toxicological Methods. 2021;**112**:107105. DOI: 10.1016/j.vascn.2021.107105

[96] Zohn IE, Sarkar AA. The visceral yolk sac endoderm provides for absorption of nutrients to the embryo during neurulation. Birth Defects Research Part A: Clinical and Molecular Teratology. 2010;**88**(8):593-600. DOI: 10.1002/bdra.20705

[97] Bjørnstad S et al. Cracking the egg: potential of the developing chicken as a model system for nonclinical safety studies of pharmaceuticals. Journal of Pharmacology and Experimental Therapeutics. 2015;**355**(3):386-396. DOI: 10.1124/jpet.115.227025

[98] Aden P et al. Low-potency glucocorticoid hydrocortisone has similar neurotoxic effects as high-potency glucocorticoid dexamethasone on neurons in the immature chicken cerebellum. Brain Research. 2008;**1236**:39-48. DOI: 10.1016/j.brainres.2008.07.095

[99] Rosa-Salva O et al. Sensitive periods for social development: interactions between predisposed and learned mechanisms. Cognition. 2021;**213**:104552. DOI: 10.1016/j.cognition.2020.104552

[100] De Haas EN et al. Prenatal and early postnatal behavioural programming in laying hens, with possible implications for the development of injurious pecking. Frontiers in Veterinary Science. 2021;**8**:693. DOI: 10.3389/fvets.2021.678500

[101] Marino L. Thinking chickens: a review of cognition, emotion, and behavior in the domestic chicken. Animal Cognition. 2017;**20**(2):127-147. DOI: 10.1007/s10071-016-1064-4

[102] Jarvis ED et al. Avian brains and a new understanding of vertebrate brain evolution. Nature Reviews Neuroscience. 2005;**6**(2):151-159. DOI: 10.1038/nrn1606

[103] Seo D, Patrick C, Kennealy P. Role of serotonin and dopamine system interactions in the neurobiology of impulsive aggression and its comorbidity with other clinical disorders. Aggression and Violent Behavior. 2008;**13**(5):383-395. DOI: 10.1016/j.avb.2008.06.003

[104] Daigle C et al. Individual consistency of feather pecking behavior in laying hens: once a feather pecker always a feather pecker? Frontiers in Veterinary Science. 2015;**2**:6. DOI: 10.3389/fvets.2015.00006

[105] Dennis RL, Fahey AG, Cheng H-w. Alterations to embryonic serotonin change aggression and fearfulness. Aggressive Behavior. 2013;**39**(2):91-98. DOI: 10.1002/ab.21459

[106] Dennis R, Cheng H-w. The dopaminergic system and aggression in laying hens. Poultry Science. 2011;**90**(11):2440-2448. DOI: 10.3382/ps.2011-01513

[107] Cheng H-w, Muir W. Chronic social stress differentially regulates neuroendocrine responses in laying hens: II. Genetic basis of adrenal responses under three different social conditions. Psychoneuroendocrinology. 2004;**29**(7):961-971. DOI: 10.1016/j.psyneuen.2003.09.002

[108] Antila H et al. Bullying involvement in relation to personality disorders: a prospective follow-up of 508 inpatient adolescents. European Child & Adolescent Psychiatry. 2017;**26**(7):779-789. DOI: 10.1007/s00787-017-0946-6

[109] Johnson K. Gut microbiome composition and diversity are related to human personality traits. Human Microbiome Journal. 2020;**15**:100069. DOI: 10.1016/j.humic.2019.100069

[110] Saffarian A et al. Crypt-and mucosa-associated core microbiotas in humans and their alteration in colon cancer patients. MBio. 2019;**10**(4):e01315-e01319. DOI: 10.1128/mBio.01315-19

[111] Mondo E et al. Gut microbiome structure and adrenocortical activity

in dogs with aggressive and phobic behavioral disorders. Heliyon. 2020;**6**(1):e03311. DOI: 10.1016/j.heliyon.2020.e03311

[112] Andoh A et al. Comparison of the gut microbial community between obese and lean peoples using 16S gene sequencing in a Japanese population. Journal of Clinical Biochemistry and Nutrition. 2016;**59**(1):65-70. DOI: 10.3164/jcbn.15-152

[113] Chen J et al. Sex differences in gut microbiota in patients with major depressive disorder. Neuropsychiatric Disease and Treatment. 2018;**14**:647-655. DOI: 10.2147/ndt.S159322

[114] Knack JM, Jensen-Campbell LA, Baum A. Worse than sticks and stones? Bullying is associated with altered HPA axis functioning and poorer health. Brain and Cognition. 2011;77(2):183-190. DOI: 10.1016/j.bandc.2011.06.011

[115] Berthoud H-R, Albaugh VL, Neuhuber WL. Gut-brain communication and obesity: understanding functions of the vagus nerve. Journal of Clinical Investigation. 2021;**131**(10):e143770. DOI: 10.1172/JCI143770

Section 3

# Cognitive Behavioral Therapy

Chapter 5

# Cognitive Behavioral Therapy in Panic Disorder

*Yavuz Yilmaz and Cicek Hocaoglu*

## Abstract

Panic disorder is an anxiety disorder characterized by panic attacks involving sudden, intense, unexpected, and recurrent fear and worry about possible future attacks. Cognitive behavioral therapy for panic disorder, which requires effective treatment, is a method that has been shown to be useful in various studies. In this section, we aimed to review the cognitive behavioral therapy applied for panic disorder. First of all, information about the definition, epidemiology, and clinical presentation and treatment options of panic disorder will be given. Then, in accordance with the main purpose of the section, the assumptions and methods of cognitive behavioral therapy for panic disorder will be explained. Finally, studies showing the effectiveness of cognitive behavioral therapy in panic disorder will be reviewed.

**Keywords:** panic disorder, cognitive behavioral therapy, treatment, breathing techniques, cognitive restructuring

## 1. Introduction

Panic disorder (PD) is a chronic psychiatric disorder characterized by unexpectedly recurring panic attacks. A panic attack is a period of intense fear that begins suddenly and lasts from a few minutes to an hour. Panic attacks can be observed in many different psychiatric and medical disorders. Patients with panic disorder experience anxiety about future attacks, for a month or longer. They exhibit recurrent untriggered panic attacks or behavioral changes related to attacks (avoiding certain situations and having repeated medical examinations) [1]. Panic attacks in PD often occur without any previous symptoms and intense physical symptoms (i.e. rapid heart rate, shortness of breath, dizziness, numbness, and tremor) and cognitive symptoms (i.e. loss of control and fear of death) are observed during the attacks. Since the attacks occur unexpectedly and cannot be controlled, the distress caused by panic attacks increases [2].

In the general population, about a quarter of people with panic disorder also have agoraphobia. The lifetime prevalence of panic disorder is 3.7% without agoraphobia and 1.1% with agoraphobia [3]. Panic attacks are more common than panic disorders and one-third of individuals experience panic attacks at some point in their lives [3–5]. PD is a picture that can show a chronic course and symptoms can recur over time [1]. In a study that followed individuals with anxiety disorder for 12 years, it was reported that the recurrence rate of PD was 56% [6]. It is observed that recurrence rate increased when sub-threshold symptoms were included [7]. In addition to the recurrence of panic symptoms, other anxiety disorders may develop over time [8]. Panic disorder can lead to significant deterioration in the social and occupational functionality of individuals, worsening of their physical health, and a significant decrease in their quality of life [9, 10].

Three types of interventions are recommended for the treatment of individuals with panic disorder. Among these interventions, psychotherapy has been proved to have the longest duration of action and followed by pharmacological therapy and self-help. Cognitive behavioral therapy (CBT) is a form of psychological treatment that has been shown to be effective for PD and it is recommended in the guidelines [11–13].

In this section, application of CBT in PB will be discussed in detail.

## 2. Cognitive behavioral therapy in panic disorder

In panic disorder, CBT is the most extensively supported psychosocial intervention method by clinical research. The aim of an effective PD treatment is not only to reduce the frequency and severity of panic attacks but also to reduce avoidance and anticipatory anxiety and to reach the patient's level of functionality before the disorder. CBT, which has been shown to be effective in achieving these goals with evidence-based data, is at least as effective as drug treatments in the treatment of PD. Another important advantage of this treatment is that it is effective in reducing recurrences. As shown in many studies, CBT is the only first-line treatment modality for PD, apart from drug treatments [14–16]. In addition, it is also an effective therapeutic approach for a significant number of patients who refuse to use medication.

From a cognitive and behavioral point of view, the disorder can be conceptualized as intense fear caused by bodily sensations, especially autonomic arousal symptoms, in individuals with psychological and genetic predispositions [17, 18]. It usually develops suddenly, without an identifiable threat [18, 19]. After a sudden panic attack, the person may start to worry about following panic attacks and focus more on the somatic symptoms of panic attacks [20–22]. During a panic attack, patients experience physical symptoms including restlessness, shortness of breath, chest tightness, palpitation, sweating, dizziness, numbness, and tingling. The patients interpret the panic attack as having a heart attack, paralysis, fainting, losing control or going crazy, and often dying. These comments and fears form the cognitive symptom pattern of the attack and increase the patient's state of restlessness or anxiety [23, 24]. Panic attacks can trigger some active avoidance actions. Patients try to stay away from situations, places, or events that may cause problems in order to avoid the anxiety caused by the panic attack and to protect themselves. This avoidance behavior may turn out to be quite severe from time to time, and patients may experience a panic attack when they encounter the avoided situation or event [23]. Agoraphobia, which is one of these avoidance behaviors, is defined as the fear or avoidance of some situations or places (i.e. waiting in line, crowds, being alone at home, shopping malls, driving, restaurants, movie theaters, large and open spaces, etc.) in which the person thinks it may be difficult to escape or help may not be available or they feel incompetent or embarrassed. For the first time, agoraphobia was included as an independent diagnosis separate from panic disorder in the DSM-5 [1].

CBT yields better results in individuals who have good problem-solving skills, are willing to solve problems, and have high motivation. Chronic stressors or problems regarding workplace, interpersonal relationships, financial conditions, and other intervening medical conditions may exacerbate the symptoms of the disease [25]. These conditions may make it difficult for the patient to comply with the therapy and drug treatment may be required when needed.

## 2.1 Evaluation

Before CBT, the patient should be evaluated in detail. The medical and psychiatric history of the patient should be taken in detail and substance-related conditions should be questioned for the diagnosis. Panic symptoms (palpitations, sweating, shortness of breath or difficulty breathing, chest pain or tightness, dizziness, paresthesias, abdominal pain, nausea, depersonalization, derealization, fear of death, and fear of losing control or going crazy) should be described in detail; the type, location, severity, and intensity of symptoms should be questioned. In addition, the beginning of the symptoms, whether there is any triggering factor, how long it takes to peak, and how long it lasts should be questioned. It also should be questioned whether the symptoms impair the person's functionality, cause any avoidance behavior, or create anticipatory anxiety. It should be noted that panic attacks can also be seen in many medical conditions. For this reason, a detailed medical history should be taken and supported by laboratory tests when necessary. Cardiovascular diseases (arrhythmia, hypertension, angina, congestive heart failure, anemia, mitral valve prolapse), respiratory system diseases (asthma, COPD, pulmonary emboli, etc.), endocrine disorders (hyperthyroidism, DM, cushing's syndrome, pheochromocytoma, etc.), neurological diseases (SVO, meniere, epilepsy, etc.), and drug changes (change in drug dose or addition of drugs such as theophylline, amphetamines, antihistamines, and steroids) should be evaluated. Psychiatric history should be taken in detail, and psychiatric conditions with panic attacks or psychiatric conditions that may accompany PD (such as anxiety disorders, trauma history, and substance use) should be questioned. In addition, the family history of a psychiatric disease, especially anxiety disorder, and the presence of a recent psychosocial stressor should be questioned.

Evaluation tools can be used for diagnosis and to monitor response to treatment. The gold standard instrument is the Panic Disorder Severity Scale [26]. It is a seven-item scale that questions the basic characteristics of the disorder such as attack frequency, attack intensity, anticipatory anxiety, phobic avoidance, avoidance of bodily sensations, and impaired functionality. The scale is widely used and has good reliability and validity.

The main purpose of therapy is to reduce reactivity to panic-related sensations, to develop alternative thoughts instead of catastrophic interpretations, to eliminate avoidance and safety behaviors, and to strengthen the ability to tolerate anxiety [27].

## 2.2 CBT techniques

### *2.2.1 Psychoeducation*

The treatment begins with psychoeducation, in which the general appearance of panic disorder and agoraphobia, how it begins, why panic and anxiety originate, and the cycle formed by physical, cognitive, and behavioral components are explained [28]. Psychoeducation usually continues throughout the therapy. Explaining the physiological changes that occur during a panic attack and describing the psychophysiology of the fight-or-flight response is part of the education. By emphasizing that the physiological changes that develop during anxiety serve to adapt, it is aimed to correct the misconceptions, common myths, and false beliefs about panic and panic symptoms that contribute to anxiety. The physical symptoms of anxiety are often not known by the patients, and the physical symptoms experienced during intense anxiety can be quite frightening for the patient. A detailed explanation regarding how the somatic symptoms develop and these symptoms are caused by anxiety can relieve the patient. Written documents such as booklets describing the bodily symptoms of anxiety and how to deal with them can be delivered to the patients.

### *2.2.2 Self-monitoring*

The patient is asked to keep a record of the attacks and daily mood throughout the therapy with the aim of observing himself correctly [28]. Self-monitoring is introduced in the first session of the treatment and continued throughout the entire treatment. It involves continuous assessment of changes in panic, anxiety, and avoidance, promoting self-awareness and acting as a therapeutic tool. The patient is asked to keep at least two self-monitoring records and is monitored while keeping a self-monitoring record. The first record is the panic attack record, which will be filled after each panic attack, and includes clues, the most distressing situations, symptoms, thoughts, and behaviors. The second record is the daily mood record, which is filled in at the end of the day and includes general and average levels of anxiety and depression. Apart from these two records, the patient may also be asked to keep a record of daily activities and avoided situations.

### *2.2.3 Breathing techniques*

During anxiety, people's breathing can accelerate. This can range from a less intense and prolonged state that can cause bodily discomfort to a severe state that can lead to a panic attack. The patients are taught correct breathing techniques in order to teach them to control their breathing when they are panicked. They are trained for slowing down their breathing and try to stay in control and calm. Breathing techniques include slow and abdominal breathing exercises. Applying these techniques regularly is very important even when the patients are calm. Applying these techniques only when the anxiety and stress level is very high (during a panic attack) may cause the patients to think that the technique does not provide enough benefit and, therefore, does not work for them [29, 30]. In order to teach the breathing techniques to the patient correctly and to make them get used to these techniques, it may be required to apply them for 5–10 minutes a day.

Breathing techniques [31]:

- Sit comfortably or lie in bed (you can close your eyes if you prefer).
- Release your muscles as much as possible.
- Breathe in through your nose in four seconds.
- Hold the air you breathe in for two seconds.
- Release your breath through your mouth, spreading it over six seconds.

- Take a short break and inhale again through your nose for four seconds, hold for two seconds and then exhale for six seconds.
- Keep trying.

Although breathing exercises can sometimes be part of treatment, it is not considered an essential part of therapy unless there is an obvious tendency to hyperventilation, since they can become an anxiety avoidance strategy [32].

*2.2.4 Progressive muscle relaxation exercises*

There are many different relaxation techniques. In the following lines, progressive muscle relaxation, which is a type of somatic coping skill that involve the patient to contract and relax the muscles in certain parts of the body, will be discussed. The progressive muscle relaxation was first described by Jacobson in 1934. It is a method that allows the entire body to be relaxed by relaxation of large muscle groups in the body, voluntarily and regularly. It is a convenient treatment method for individuals with high anxiety levels and overly nervous. It teaches us to differentiate between the systematic tension and release of various muscle groups by being aware of the resulting sensation of tension and relaxation. It almost completely eliminates muscle contractions and creates a feeling of deep relaxation [33, 34].

Progressive muscle relaxation exercises [31]:

Sit comfortably, but avoid a position that will cause you to sleep. Slow down your breathing rate. When you are ready, you will stretch your first muscle. Keep stretching for five seconds, making sure to stretch each muscle group until you feel the tightness (but not pain); then you need to relax the same muscle group and feel this relaxation state for ten seconds. You will repeat this twice for the same muscle. Try to feel the difference between your muscle being tense and relaxed.

- First, clench your fist to stretch your right hand and lower arm, hold for five seconds, then release, and feel this relaxed state in your lower arm for ten seconds. Then repeat it again
- Now, to stretch your right upper arm, bring your lower forearm close to your shoulder, inflating the biceps. Feel the tension for five seconds and release and feel the relaxed state for ten seconds. Then, repeat the same action.

Continue stretching and relaxing exercises with these muscle groups:

- Left hand and lower forearm
- Left upper arm
- Forehead (raise your eyebrows as high as possible to make you look surprised)
- Eyes and cheeks (Tighten firmly)
- Mouth and jaw (Open your mouth wide as when yawning)

- Neck (Be slow and careful while tensing the muscles here. Lie face down if possible and raise your head as if you are looking at a point on the ceiling)
- Shoulders (tense your muscles as you bring your shoulders closer to your ears)
- Back (Push your shoulders back as if trying to bring them together)
- Chest and stomach (Breathe deeply so that your chest and stomach swell)
- Hips (Tighten the muscles in your hips)
- Right upper leg - Right lower leg (Do this slowly and carefully to avoid cramping. Tense your leg by stretching your toes toward you)
- Right foot: stretch your toes in the opposite direction
- Left upper leg
- Left lower leg
- Left foot

### *2.2.5 Cognitive restructuring*

Cognitive restructuring is one of the important components of therapy. The aim of cognitive restructuring is to be able to produce realistic alternatives by recognizing faulty cognitions in the form of catastrophizing and overestimating the threat by questioning their validity [28]. In this intervention, the effect of thoughts on emotions is explained, and thoughts in anxious moments are captured and handled; however it is not aimed to reduce anxiety, but to change the thoughts that cause it. For this purpose, it is necessary to detect and evaluate the negative automatic thoughts of the patient. Negative automatic thoughts are patterns of thinking that lead individuals to judge themselves, external world, and the future negatively [35]. Some methods including direct questions, detection of automatic thoughts by guided exploration, worst-case scenario technique, recording thoughts accompanied by behavior experiment, and automatic thought recording can be applied to detect and evaluate these thoughts. In "direct questions" method, the patient can be questioned about what thoughts go through his/her mind when he/she has a panic attack. For example, questions such as "What was going through your mind when you felt your heart speed up?" "If we had the chance to read your mind at that time, what would we see?" can be asked of the patient who had a panic attack. Detection of automatic thoughts by guided exploration is a method that can be applied to the patients who have difficulty remembering automatic thoughts. The situation in which the patient is experiencing distress is handled, it is tried to catch the moment when intense anxiety/panic symptoms appear, the factors accompanying intense anxiety/panic symptoms are handled and the thought is tried to be reached. Worst-case scenario technique is effectively used in patients who have difficulty capturing automatic thoughts. In this method, it is aimed to detect automatic thoughts by asking the question "What is the worst thing that could happen?" considering the environment, situation, and symptoms. In recording thoughts accompanied by behavior experiment method, the patients may be asked to experience a distressing situation and record the thoughts in their minds. For example, the patients can be asked to breathe quickly as they were experiencing complaints similar to the panic attacks and record their thoughts in their minds during that experience. In automatic thought recording method, the patients are informed about automatic thoughts and then they are asked to keep a record of these thoughts by using an automatic thought registration form. Once negative automatic thoughts are identified, the next thing to do is to focus on these thoughts. It is more accurate to evaluate how to comply or not these thoughts with the reality rather than characterizing negative automatic thoughts as right or wrong. The aim is to detect the negative automatic thoughts that do not fully comply with reality and to shake the belief in these thoughts by using different techniques. As the intensity of the patient's belief in these thoughts decreases, the feeling of discomfort caused by these thoughts will also decrease. Continuous examination of negative automatic thoughts has benefits such as increasing awareness of the patient, decreasing the frequency of negative thoughts, and enabling the patients to produce alternatives when these thoughts come to their minds. The methods including examining evidence, finding cognitive distortions, the double standard technique, and alternative explanations can be used to evaluate negative automatic thoughts. Evidence review is one of the reality-based techniques in cognitive restructuring and it is based on the examination of evidence that may or may not support the reality of negative automatic thinking. This approach is aimed to raise a suspicion against this thought in the patients and to encourage a more realistic perspective by examining the evidence supporting or not supporting negative thinking. Starting with the evidence supporting negative thinking can be helpful in avoiding the patients to feel disapproved and encouraging them to be critical of their own thinking. The patients will not have much difficulty finding evidence to support it thanks to their strong belief in negative thinking. However, the therapists should be more helpful to the patients experiencing difficulty in finding counter-evidence. Automatic thoughts are also called cognitive distortions or cognitive errors. In recent years, cognitive behavioral therapists prefer the term "error" to the term "distortion" [36]. It is not necessary to investigate cognitive distortions in CBT; however, this investigation may benefit the patients in finding and coping with negative automatic thoughts. In finding cognitive distortions, the concept of cognitive distortion should be explained to the patient theoretically, thought distortions should be shared with the patient, and it should be detected which one of the patient's negative thoughts corresponds with cognitive distortion. Then, the patient may be asked to find the cognitive distortions in the negative automatic thoughts that he/she will record himself/herself. The main purpose of this approach is to provide the patient with the chance to look at and examine their own thoughts from the outside. At this point, the most common cognitive distortions, including catastrophizing, mind-reading, fortune-telling, all-or-nothing thinking, ignoring the positive, overgeneralizing, and personalizing, can be explained to the patients. In the double standard technique, the patients are asked what a friend experiencing similar situation would do in order to reveal the nonobjective self-evaluation of the patients. Since it provides the opportunity to look at the situation from someone else's perspective, it provides the chance to make more objective and more realistic evaluations. It can be in the form of asking questions directly, or it can be done through a scenario. In alternative explanations technique, the patients may be asked questions about what else the situation they are experiencing may mean or in what other situations it can be experienced, or how they would interpret the situation if it would happen to someone else.

### *2.2.6 Exposure*

Exposure is the main application of CBT for PD and it aims to change the fear of the patients conditioned to certain situations and contexts by exposure to real life (in vivo) and to change the fear of bodily sensations with internal (interoceptive) exposure [28]. *In vivo* exposure involves repeated and gradual exposure to agoraphobic situations in the real life. It is aimed to eliminate avoidance, reduce catastrophic thoughts, and ultimately reduce fear and anxiety. Although there is evidence to suggest that non-gradual exposure to intense anxiety-provoking situations may also be beneficial, it has been observed that gradual exposure, starting with less anxiety-provoking situations, yields better results [37]. In this case, it is recommended to list the situations that the patient avoids and start with exposure to a moderately irritating situation. The aim is to expose the patient to these situations or environments until the level of anxiety decreases. Patients may exhibit safety behaviors, including avoidance. These behaviors involve the actions that a person does to prevent the disaster she or he fears. The patients may avoid environments that they think will trigger the attack or may display actions in order to eliminate the symptoms. These actions include moving slowly for fear of having a heart attack, avoiding going to places far from the hospital, checking the presence of other people around, and paying attention to the entrances and exits in closed areas. Safety behaviors may have a short-term calming effect in PD patients, however, these actions cause increased anxiety and continued anxiety in the long term. *In vivo* exposure also serves to reduce belief and confidence in safety behaviors. *In vivo* exposure can initially be done under the supervision of a therapist, then self-administered exposure assignments can be given between sessions.

The aim of interoceptive exposure is to sustain the feared physical sensations with sufficient duration and intensity by stimulating them and to make the patients experience the extinction of the resulting anxiety response. The most used method in PD is hyperventilation exercise. The patients artificially induce a panic attack. By staying in that state, they can realize that this is not actually a sign of a bad disease, but just a natural reaction of the body. They observe that this attack can be easily extinguished by breathing exercises. In this way, the belief that the symptoms patients experience are under their own control is reinforced [38]. Methods that trigger bodily symptoms such as caffeine consumption and exercise are other stimuli that can be used for interoceptive exposure. First, it is applied under the supervision of the therapist during the session, then the patient is asked to apply it himself/herself between the sessions. In the next step, *in vivo* exposure and interoceptive exposure can be combined. Some patients should be paid attention during the exposure to situations. In patients with cardiac (such as arrhythmia) and respiratory (such as asthma) problems, exposure should be avoided or gradual exposure should be applied since the patients will experience intense anxiety during exposure.

### *2.2.7 Preventing recurrence*

The final stage of CBT is prevention of recurrence. In this stage, it is important to inform patients that even if they have improved, they may experience anxiety symptoms again in the future and have panic attacks again. It should be explained that this situation is not a treatment failure, it is a possible situation due to the nature of the disease, and in this case, they may need to use coping skills again.

### 2.3 Number of sessions

Sessions can be administered one to one or in small groups. Each session lasts 60–120 minutes and 10–20 treatment sessions are applied weekly. Positive results have also been reported in patients who received one, four, six, or seven sessions or in those who were treated intensively for two days [39–42].

### 2.4 Concomitant diseases and indicators of response to treatment

A significant proportion of those with anxiety disorders meets the criteria for at least one other disorder. The most common accompanying diagnoses include anxiety disorders, mood disorders, substance use disorders, and somatoform disorders [43, 44]. This raises the question of whether the presence of an accompanying psychiatric disorder affects the treatment results. While it has been observed that comorbid anxiety disorders and mood disorders do not reduce the effectiveness of CBT, the effect of comorbid depression on the effectiveness of CBT is controversial [45–50]. It is thought that the presence of a diagnosis of comorbid personality disorder may be associated with a poor response to CBT and may require a longer CBT regimen [51, 52]. Whether medical comorbid conditions affect the effectiveness of CBT has not been studied in detail, but cardiac (such as arrhythmias) and respiratory problems (such as asthma) may cause a decrease in recovery rates. The benefit obtained from CBT was found to be related to the compliance of the patients with the homework given [53].

### 2.5 Effectivity

Meta-analyses have shown that CBT generally provides significant improvement and regression in symptoms in individuals with anxiety disorder and PD [53–57]. In a meta-analysis of five randomized, placebo-controlled studies on a patient group with panic disorder/agoraphobia, CBT was found to be effective compared to placebo or psychological control [58]. This finding supports the findings of previous meta-analyses with similar results [59–61]. It has been reported that although recurrence may develop over time, the effectiveness of CBT continues, there is no significant decrease in effectiveness in 6 and 12-month follow-ups, and the recurrence rate is half that of pharmacotherapy [15, 59, 60, 62]. Although CBT gives positive results in many patients, there are cases where it may be insufficient. In a study in which the long-term effectiveness of CBT was monitored in patients with PD, it was reported that panic-related symptoms showed a fluctuating course, the treatment response was insufficient, only 48% of the patients had a significant reduction in panic, anxiety, and avoidance symptoms, and some of the patients (27%) sought different methods for panic symptoms due to inadequate treatment response [62]. The rates of compliance and continuation of the treatment also vary. In a clinical study, the mean quit rate was reported to be 19% in patients who started CBT for panic disorder/agoraphobia [60].

## 3. Conclusions

Panic disorder is a chronic psychiatric disorder characterized by unexpectedly recurring panic attacks. A panic attack is a period of intense fear that begins suddenly and lasts from a few minutes to an hour. The lifetime prevalence of panic disorder is 3.7% without agoraphobia and 1.1% with agoraphobia. Panic attacks are more common than panic disorders. One-third of individuals experience panic attacks at some point in their lives.

When the panic disorder model of cognitive behavioral therapy is examined, it is seen that panic disorder begins as a catastrophizing of various bodily sensations and intellectual activities and intense anxiety. The individual determines various strategies in order to not experience this intense anxiety again. However, inaccurate strategies cause more anxiety instead of protecting the individual from anxiety. These coping strategies involve avoidance of certain places and situations where there is a threat of experiencing a panic attack and exhibiting certain safety behaviors. Coping strategies may help to alleviate anxiety for a short time, but in the long term, they cause the disorder to be sustained and become chronic.

Panic attacks begin suddenly without a reason and quickly become severe. During an attack, intense somatic symptoms are experienced and the patients interpret these symptoms with a catastrophizing way of thinking. They think that they have a heart attack, that they will lose control, and even that they will die. This situation continues in a vicious circle and causes anxiety to increase gradually. In cognitive behavioral therapy, a treatment protocol was determined based on this panic disorder model. One of the most important components of treatment is psychoeducation, that is, explaining what a panic attack is and the nature of what is experienced. Psychoeducation is aimed to explain that panic attacks are not actually dangerous, but only a natural reaction of the body to anxiety. The aim of self-monitoring is to observe one's self correctly. Strategies for coping with anxiety such as breathing techniques and progressive muscle relaxation exercises are taught. Cognitive restructuring, which is one of the important components of the CBT, is aimed to realize the faulty cognitions in the form of catastrophizing and overestimating the threat, question their validity, and produce realistic alternatives to these cognitions. Another important component of treatment is exposure. It is very important for the treatment that the individual is systematically exposed to the situations and places they avoid, and in this way making the patients realize that the feared places and situations do not really pose a threat.

## Conflict of interest

The authors declare no conflict of interest.

## Author details

Yavuz Yilmaz[1]* and Cicek Hocaoglu[2]

1 Faculty of Medicine, Department of Psychiatry, Cumhuriyet University, Sivas, Turkey

2 Faculty of Medicine, Department of Psychiatry, Recep Tayip Erdogan University, Rize, Turkey

*Address all correspondence to: dr.yavuzz@hotmail.com

## References


[1] American Psychiatric Association. Diagnostic and Statistical Manual of Mental Disorders, Fifth Edition (DSM-5). Arlington, VA: American Psychiatric Association; 2013

[2] Wolf AW, Goldfried MR. Clinical experiences in using cognitive-behavior therapy to treat panic disorder. Behavior Therapy. 2014;**45**(1):36-46. DOI: 10.1016/j.beth.2013.10.002

[3] Kessler RC, Chiu WT, Jin R, Ruscio AM, Shear K, Walters EE. The epidemiology of panic attacks, panic disorder, and agoraphobia in the National Comorbidity Survey Replication. Archives of General Psychiatry. 2006;**63**(4):415-424. DOI: 10.1001/archpsyc.63.4.415

[4] Katon W, Vitaliano PP, Russo J, Jones M, Anderson K, Panic disorder. Spectrum of severity and somatization. The Journal of Nervous and Mental Disease. 1987;**175**(1):12-19

[5] Smoller JW, Pollack MH, Wassertheil-Smoller S, et al. Prevalence and correlates of panic attacks in postmenopausal women: Results from an ancillary study to the Women's Health Initiative. Archives of Internal Medicine. 2003;**163**(17):2041-2050. DOI: 10.1001/archinte.163.17.2041

[6] Bruce SE, Yonkers KA, Otto MW, et al. Influence of psychiatric comorbidity on recovery and recurrence in generalized anxiety disorder, social phobia, and panic disorder: A 12-year prospective study. The American Journal of Psychiatry. 2005;**162**(6):1179-1187. DOI: 10.1176/appi.ajp.162.6.1179

[7] Nay W, Brown R, Roberson-Nay R. Longitudinal course of panic disorder with and without agoraphobia using the National Epidemiologic Survey on Alcohol and Related Conditions (NESARC). Psychiatry Research. 2013;**208**(1):54-61. DOI: 10.1016/j.psychres.2013.03.006

[8] Scholten WD, Batelaan NM, van Balkom AJ, Wjh Penninx B, Smit JH, van Oppen P. Recurrence of anxiety disorders and its predictors. Journal of Affective Disorders. 2013;**147**(1-3):180-185. DOI: 10.1016/j.jad.2012.10.031

[9] Chambless DL, Milrod B, Porter E, et al. Prediction and moderation of improvement in cognitive-behavioral and psychodynamic psychotherapy for panic disorder. Journal of Consulting and Clinical Psychology. 2017;**85**(8):803-813. DOI: 10.1037/ccp0000224

[10] Fava GA, Rafanelli C, Ottolini F, Ruini C, Cazzaro M, Grandi S. Psychological well-being and residual symptoms in remitted patients with panic disorder and agoraphobia. Journal of Affective Disorders. 2001;**65**(2):185-190. DOI: 10.1016/s0165-0327(00)00267-6

[11] Practice guideline for the treatment of patients with panic disorder. Work Group on Panic Disorder. American Psychiatric Association. The American Journal of Psychiatry. 1998;**155**(Suppl. 5):1-34

[12] Royal Australian and New Zealand College of Psychiatrists Clinical Practice Guidelines Team for Panic Disorder and Agoraphobia. Australian and New Zealand clinical practice guidelines for the treatment of panic disorder and agoraphobia. The Australian and New Zealand Journal of Psychiatry. 2003;**37**(6):641-656. DOI: 10.1080/j.1440-1614.2003.01254.x

[13] NICE. Generalised Anxiety Disorder and Panic Disorder in Adults: Management. London: National Institute for Health and Care Excellence (NICE); July 2019

[14] Bruinsma A, Kampman M, Exterkate CC, Hendriks GJ. Een verkennende studie naar blended cognitieve gedragstherapie voor paniek-stoornis: Resultaten en patiëntervaringen [An exploratory study of 'blended' cognitive behavioural therapy (CBT) for patients with a panic disorder: Results and patients' experiences]. Tijdschrift voor Psychiatrie. 2016;**58**(5):361-370

[15] Butler AC, Chapman JE, Forman EM, Beck AT. The empirical status of cognitive-behavioral therapy: A review of meta-analyses. Clinical Psychology Review. 2006;**26**(1):17-31. DOI: 10.1016/j.cpr.2005.07.003

[16] Otto MW, Pollack MH, Dowd SM, et al. Randomized trial of d-cycloserine enhancement of cognitive-behavioral therapy for panic disorder. Depression and Anxiety. 2016;**33**(8):737-745. DOI: 10.1002/da.22531

[17] Barlow D. Anxiety and Its Disorders: The Nature and Treatment of Anxiety and Panic. 2nd ed. New York: Guilford Press; 2002

[18] Craske M. The Origins of Phobias and Anxiety Disorders: Why More Women than Men? Oxford: Elsevier Science; 2003

[19] Barlow D. Office-based behavioural treatment of panic attack. In: Panic Disorder: Relative Merits of Pharmacotherapy and Psychotherapy. Ontario: The Medicine Group; 1988. p. 6

[20] Hayward C, Killen JD, Kraemer HC, Taylor CB. Predictors of panic attacks in adolescents. Journal of the American Academy of Child and Adolescent Psychiatry. 2000;**39**(2):207-214. DOI: 10.1097/00004583-200002000-00021

[21] Ehlers A. A 1-year prospective study of panic attacks: Clinical course and factors associated with maintenance. Journal of Abnormal Psychology. 1995;**104**(1):164-172. DOI: 10.1037//0021-843x.104.1.164

[22] Schmidt NB, Lerew DR, Jackson RJ. The role of anxiety sensitivity in the pathogenesis of panic: Prospective evaluation of spontaneous panic attacks during acute stress. Journal of Abnormal Psychology. 1997;**106**(3):355-364. DOI: 10.1037//0021-843x.106.3.355

[23] American Psychiatric Association. Diagnostic and Statistical Manual of Mental Disorders fourth edition (DSM–IV). Washington DC: American Psychiatric Association; 1994

[24] Aronson TA, Logue CM. Phenomenology of panic attacks: A descriptive study of panic disorder patients' self-reports. The Journal of Clinical Psychiatry. 1988;**49**(1):8-13

[25] Sanderson WC, Bruce TJ. Causes and management of treatment-resistant panic disorder and agoraphobia: A survey of expert therapists. Cognitive and Behavioral Practice. 2007;**14**(1):26-35

[26] Shear MK, Brown TA, Barlow DH, et al. Multicenter collaborative panic disorder severity scale. The American Journal of Psychiatry. 1997;**154**(11):1571-1575. DOI: 10.1176/ajp.154.11.1571

[27] Clark DA, Beck AT. Cognitive Therapy of Anxiety Disorders: Science and Practice. New York: Guilford Press; 2011

[28] Craske MG, ve Barlow, D. H. Panic disorder and agoraphobia.

In: Barlow DH, editor. Clinical Handbook of Psychological Disorders: A Step-by-step Treatment Manual. New York: The Guilford Press; 2014. pp. 1-62

[29] Davis M, Eshelman ER, McKay M. The Relaxation and Stress Reduction Workbook. Oakland: New Harbinger Publications; 2008

[30] Barlow DH. Anxiety and Its Disorders: The Nature and Treatment of Anxiety and Panic. New York: Guilford Press; 2004

[31] Taken from the website of the Turkish Psychiatric Association. Access address: https://psychiatry.org.tr/uploadFiles/2132020115258-gevsemebrosur.pdf

[32] McCabe RE, Antony MM. Panic disorder and agoraphobia. In: Antony MM, Ledley DR, Heimberg RG, editors. Improving Outcome and Preventing Relapse in Cognitivebehavioral Therapy. New York: The Guilford Press; 2005, 2005. pp. 1-38

[33] Essa RM, Ismail NIAA, Hassan NI. Effect of progressive muscle relaxation technique on stress, anxiety, and depression after hysterectomy. Journal of Nursing Education and Practice. 2017;**7**(7):77-86

[34] McCallie MS, Blum CM, Hood CJ. Progressive muscle relaxation. Journal of Human Behavior in the Social Environment. 2006;**13**(1):51-66

[35] Coyne JC, Gotlib IH. The role of cognition in depression: A critical appraisal. Psychological Bulletin. 1983;**94**(3):472-505

[36] Özdel K, Taymur I, Guriz SO, Tulaci RG, Kuru E, Turkcapar MH. Measuring cognitive errors using the Cognitive Distortions Scale (CDS): Psychometric properties in clinical and non-clinical samples. PLoS One. 2014;**9**(8):e105956

[37] Fiegenbaum W. Long-term efficacy of ungraded versus graded massed exposure in agoraphobics. In: Panic and Phobias 2. Berlin, Heidelberg: Springer; 1988. pp. 83-88

[38] Bouchard S, Gauthier J, Laberge B, French D, Pelletier MH, Godbout C. Exposure versus cognitive restructuring in the treatment of panic disorder with agoraphobia. Behaviour Research and Therapy. 1996;**34**(3):213-224. DOI: 10.1016/0005-7967(95)00077-1

[39] Lessard MJ, Marchand A, Pelland MÈ, et al. Comparing two brief psychological interventions to usual care in panic disorder patients presenting to the emergency department with chest pain. Behavioural and Cognitive Psychotherapy. 2012;**40**(2):129-147. DOI: 10.1017/S1352465811000506

[40] Craske MG, Maidenberg E, Bystritsky A. Brief cognitive-behavioral versus nondirective therapy for panic disorder. Journal of Behavior Therapy and Experimental Psychiatry. 1995;**26**(2):113-120. DOI: 10.1016/0005-7916(95)00003-i

[41] Clark DM, Salkovskis PM, Hackmann A, Wells A, Ludgate J, Gelder M. Brief cognitive therapy for panic disorder: A randomized controlled trial. Journal of Consulting and Clinical Psychology. 1999;**67**(4):583-589. DOI: 10.1037//0022-006x.67.4.583

[42] Deacon B, Abramowitz J. A pilot study of two-day cognitive-behavioral therapy for panic disorder. Behaviour Research and Therapy. 2006;**44**(6):807-817. DOI: 10.1016/j.brat.2005.05.008

[43] Kessler RC, Nelson CB, McGonagle KA, Liu J, Swartz M,

Blazer DG. Comorbidity of DSM-III-R major depressive disorder in the general population: Results from the US National Comorbidity Survey. The British Journal of Psychiatry. Supplement. 1996;**30**:17-30

[44] Brown TA, Chorpita BF, Barlow DH. Structural relationships among dimensions of the DSM-IV anxiety and mood disorders and dimensions of negative affect, positive affect, and autonomic arousal. Journal of Abnormal Psychology. 1998;**107**(2):179-192. DOI: 10.1037//0021-843x.107.2.179

[45] Brown TA, Antony MM, Barlow DH. Diagnostic comorbidity in panic disorder: Effect on treatment outcome and course of comorbid diagnoses following treatment. Journal of Consulting and Clinical Psychology. 1995;**63**(3):408-418. DOI: 10.1037//0022-006x.63.3.408

[46] Allen L, Barlow D. Treatment of panic disorder: Outcomes and basic processes. In: Rothbaum B, editor. Pathological Anxiety: Emotional Processing in Etiology and Treatment. New York: Guilford Press; 2006. p. 166

[47] McLean PD, Woody S, Taylor S, Koch WJ. Comorbid panic disorder and major depression: Implications for cognitive-behavioral therapy. Journal of Consulting and Clinical Psychology. 1998;**66**(2):240-247. DOI: 10.1037//0022-006x.66.2.240

[48] Laberge B, Gauthier JG, Côté G, Plamondon J, Cormier HJ. Cognitive-behavioral therapy of panic disorder with secondary major depression: A preliminary investigation. Journal of Consulting and Clinical Psychology. 1993;**61**(6):1028-1037. DOI: 10.1037//0022-006x.61.6.1028

[49] Maddock RJ, Blacker KH. Response to treatment in panic disorder with associated depression. Psychopathology. 1991;**24**(1):1-6. DOI: 10.1159/000284689

[50] Wade WA, Treat TA, Stuart GL. Transporting an empirically supported treatment for panic disorder to a service clinic setting: A benchmarking strategy. Journal of Consulting and Clinical Psychology. 1998;**66**(2):231-239. DOI: 10.1037//0022-006x.66.2.231

[51] Marchand A et al. Personality disorders and the outcome of cognitive–behavioural treatment of panic disorder with agoraphobia. Canadian Journal of Behavioural Science/Revue canadienne des sciences du comportement. 1998;**30**(1):14

[52] van den Hout M, Brouwers C, Oomen J. Clinically diagnosed axis II co-morbidity and the short term outcome of CBT for axis I disorders. Clinical Psychology & Psychotherapy: An International Journal of Theory & Practice. 2006;**13**(1):56-63

[53] Kazantzis N, Ronan KR, Deane FP. Concluding causation from correlation: Comment on Burns and Spangler (2000). Journal of Consulting and Clinical Psychology. 2001;**69**(6):1079-1086. DOI: 10.1037//0022-006x.69.6.1079

[54] Pompoli A, Furukawa TA, Imai H, Tajika A, Efthimiou O, Salanti G. Psychological therapies for panic disorder with or without agoraphobia in adults: A network meta-analysis. Cochrane Database of Systematic Reviews. 2016;**4**(4):CD011004

[55] Bandelow B, Reitt M, Röver C, Michaelis S, Görlich Y, Wedekind D. Efficacy of treatments for anxiety disorders: A meta-analysis. International Clinical Psychopharmacology. 2015;**30**(4):183-192. DOI: 10.1097/YIC.0000000000000078

[56] Cuijpers P, Gentili C, Banos RM, Garcia-Campayo J, Botella C, Cristea IA. Relative effects of cognitive and behavioral therapies on generalized anxiety disorder, social anxiety disorder and panic disorder: A meta-analysis. Journal of Anxiety Disorders. 2016;**43**:79-89. DOI: 10.1016/j.janxdis.2016.09.003

[57] Watts SE, Turnell A, Kladnitski N, Newby JM, Andrews G. Treatment-as-usual (TAU) is anything but usual: A meta-analysis of CBT versus TAU for anxiety and depression. Journal of Affective Disorders. 2015;**175**:152-167. DOI: 10.1016/j.jad.2014.12.025

[58] Carpenter JK, Andrews LA, Witcraft SM, Powers MB, Smits JAJ, Hofmann SG. Cognitive behavioral therapy for anxiety and related disorders: A meta-analysis of randomized placebo-controlled trials. Depression and Anxiety. 2018;**35**(6):502-514. DOI: 10.1002/da.22728

[59] Norton PJ, Price EC. A meta-analytic review of adult cognitive-behavioral treatment outcome across the anxiety disorders. The Journal of Nervous and Mental Disease. 2007;**195**(6):521-531. DOI: 10.1097/01.nmd.0000253843.70149.9a

[60] Haby MM, Donnelly M, Corry J, Vos T. Cognitive behavioural therapy for depression, panic disorder and generalized anxiety disorder: A meta-regression of factors that may predict outcome. The Australian and New Zealand Journal of Psychiatry. 2006;**40**(1):9-19. DOI: 10.1080/j.1440-1614.2006.01736.x

[61] Vos SP, Huibers MJ, Diels L, Arntz A. A randomized clinical trial of cognitive behavioral therapy and interpersonal psychotherapy for panic disorder with agoraphobia. Psychological Medicine. 2012;**42**(12):2661-2672. DOI: 10.1017/S0033291712000876

[62] Brown TA, Barlow DH. Long-term outcome in cognitive-behavioral treatment of panic disorder: Clinical predictors and alternative strategies for assessment. Journal of Consulting and Clinical Psychology. 1995;**63**(5):754-765. DOI: 10.1037//0022-006x.63.5.754